D1570087

AIDS
IN AMERICA

our chances, our choices

AIDS
IN AMERICA

our chances, our choices

by

Robert E. Lee

The Whitston Publishing Company
Troy, New York
1987

Library of Congress Catalog Card Number 87-51105

ISBN 0-87875-355-9 (clothbound)
ISBN 0-87875-357-5 (paperbound)

Printed in the United States of America

To my family, with love . . .

Contents

Prologue

Since 1986, the Acquired Immunodeficiency Syndrome (AIDS) has become daily media grist. Stories circulate among us of "friends of friends" being afflicted and dying from AIDS, yet most of us still have had no immediate experience with the disease. Recent reports (1978 to March 1985) from the Federal Government of the potential of AIDS infection from receipt of blood through transfusion have frightened us of the hidden power of this "new invader." An uneasiness about our own fallibility is ever-so-gradually settling into our subconsciousness. The "day-light" of science, firmly rooted as our "can-do" shield, is beginning to waver.

This mystery disease, despite our fears, surely can be solved by the scientific brain trust—or can it? According to David Baltimore, AIDS expert and Nobel laureate, "It will probably be the most important public-health problem of the next decade and going into the next century."[1] His comment is representative of a growing host of normally restrained scientists. The AIDS threat "is probably more serious than has been thought" and the disease stands every chance of becoming the threat of the century.[2] Reports such as these begin to show the magnitude of concern among AIDS scientists. Imagine this possibility:

> It is the year 2001 and, although the full scientific knowledge of molecular biology has been focused on defeating AIDS since 1983, there is still no cure and no vaccine. Continuing efforts have begun to affect the nation's sexual behavior in order to reduce the risk of contracting AIDS, but that change in behavior occurred too late for millions of persons. There are now over 50 million persons seropositive (blood-testing positive) for AIDS. Nearly 1.5 million persons die this year alone from the disease. You have had someone close to you die. You know many who are infected—you may be infected. Epidemiological reports of the probable number of persons infected within 5 years by AIDS soar to perhaps 100 million persons in the United States alone.
>
> The social fabric of the nation is threatened; constitutional rights have been suspended. In some areas of the nation, marshal

> law is the order. Certain remote areas have become "AIDS-Free Zones"—those found to be infected are summarily executed by residents and Zone boundaries are patrolled by armed guards. Certain larger cities of the nation have ceased provision of municipal services by default because there is not a sufficient number of employees left alive to provide the service. Disposal of the dead is now by mass grave or bonfire. Fanatical elements of society are profligating; travel is now a risk. Wildfire rumors of conspiracy, germ-warfare, divine judgment, and apocalypse sweep the country.

Is this science fiction? Is AIDS to be "an Andromeda strain"? David Baltimore also states "The consequences already look catastrophic. A quarter of a million people with a lethal disease is catastrophic—and that's the United States only. And that's the rock-bottom projection for 1991." With cases doubling every 13 months, AIDS is certain to take its place among the ranks as one of the world's major killers. Dr. Stephen Jay Gould, a Harvard University biologist, has stated AIDS is "an issue that may rank with nuclear weaponry as the greatest danger of our era" and may be the "greatest natural tragedy" in history.[3]

AIDS is a life-threatening disease for which there is no effective cure, and the number of cases is growing exponentially. As of September 15th, 1986, there were 24,859 reported cases of AIDS in the United States and 13,689 patients had died. It was estimated that 1.5 to 2 million people were infected with the virus. By the end of 1986 about 15,000 Americans had died of the disease and it was estimated that of the 10 million people who carry the virus worldwide (then approximately 1.5 million of them in the U.S.), 25 to 30 percent would have the disease within five years. As of March 1987, U. S. figures for AIDS showed 32,000 diagnosed, 19,000 dead and an estimated 2.5 million persons infected but not yet diagnosed.

Just as sobering is the firm evidence that with the passage of time after exposure the risk of developing AIDS may actually increase, rather than decrease. Evidence in early 1987 suggested that at least 50% of AIDS-infected persons will eventually progress to the full-blown disease. Dr. Robert Redfield (Walter Reed Army Institute of Research) found that 90% of AIDS-infected persons progress from an early stage of HTLV-III infection-related symptoms to more severe forms of the disease.

In past cases epidemiologists have been able to construct mathematical models tracing probable development of a disease, but, because of the newness of AIDS, accurate modeling has yet to be accomplished. The number of variables necessary to deevelop an effective model are simply not known. However, if AIDS continues at its current rate of growth and ceases to be selective of its victim-groups, estimates quickly reveal a plague of major proportions by 2001. In that year alone, 3.5 million may be diagnosed, 50 million may be infected but not yet diagnosed, and 1.5 million may die. "If we can't make progress [against AIDS], we face the dreadful prospect of a worldwide death toll in the tens of millions a decade from now," warned Health and Human Services Secretary Otis Bowen at a recent gathering of the National Press Club. "Such earlier epidemics as typhus, small-pox and even the black death will 'look very pale by comparison'—you haven't read or heard anything yet."[4]

Factors mitigating against this scenario are equally unknown. Among questions of importance in the growth of AIDS are:

1. When did AIDS first infect mankind?
2. Where did it come from?
3. How could AIDS suddenly appear?
4. Does everyone who gets AIDS die?
5. Does everyone have an equal chance of contracting the disease?
6. How long is the incubation period before clinical symptoms appear?
7. Will the exponential growth rate continue or decline?
8. Will an effective vaccine be developed?
9. Will sufficient changes occur in the nation's sexual morality and behavior to stem AID's spread?
10. Are there any methods of spreading the disease that are not yet discovered?
11. Will the disease "run its course" in the high-risk groups or will it spread to the heterosexual community?

This disease is truly an unprecedented mystery and challenge to modern science, one potentially capable of defying solution. We, humankind, are in a contest. Will we be victorious over this disease or will it be victorious over us? This contest is time-limited. Given the worst scenario, we have 23 years until the clock runs out and the human race is decimated. Given the best scenario, within 5 to 10 years a solution will be found with a "minimum" number of casualties, i.e., 2-5 million dead in the U.S. alone. Should AIDS invade the heterosexual population of the United States as it has in central Africa, that continent may have a stark lesson to teach our country about how suddenly and inexorably the disease can erode and destroy our comfortable assumptions and familiar habits. As time passes, cumulative growth of AIDS and shifts in growth rates among infected subpopulations in the United States will continue to show us that we are not immune to the most primitive —and frightening—forces of nature.

In this book, we will examine the future of AIDS in America. Information about the scientific struggle, the potential magnitude of the disease, the social impact, and individual protection will be presented. The objective of this book is NOT sensationalism—it is a logical presentation of the potential catastrophe which may soon confront us.

Notes

[1]"Quarantining Will Help No One," an interview with AIDS expert and Nobel laureate David Baltimore, *U. S. News and World Report*, Jan.12, 1987: 70.

[2]Maddox, J. "Further Anxieties About AIDS"; *Nature*, Jan. 2, 1986: 9.

[3]Buckley, W. F. "The Buyer May Be the Smarter Person," *Moline (Illinois) Daily Dispatch*, April 28, 1987: 4.

[4]*Summit Journal*, March 1987.

A Description of the Enemy

What is Aids?

The AIDS virus, sometimes called "Human Immunodeficiency Virus" (HIV), "Human T-Cell Lymphotropic Virus-III" (HTLV-III), or "Lymphadenopathy Virus" (LAV) is an incredibly small organism, roughly 1,000 angstrom units (one ten-thousandth of a millimeter) across—just a little larger than the wavelength of red light. Neither plant nor animal, the virus particle (virion) is covered by two layers of fatty material that are stolen from the outer covering of the human host cell (T4-Lymphocyte—a white blood cell). Studding the AIDS retrovirus's surface, much like straight pins protruding from a pin cushion, are 'glycoproteins'—proteins with sugar molecule chains attached. Each glycoprotein has two components: glycoprotein-41 (gp-41)—the body of the example pin—spans the spherical surface of the virus, and glycoprotein-120 (gp-120)—the head of the example pin—extends beyond the spherical surface placed at the end of gp-41. The spherical surface covers a core made up of proteins designated protein-24 (p-24) and protein-18 (p-18).

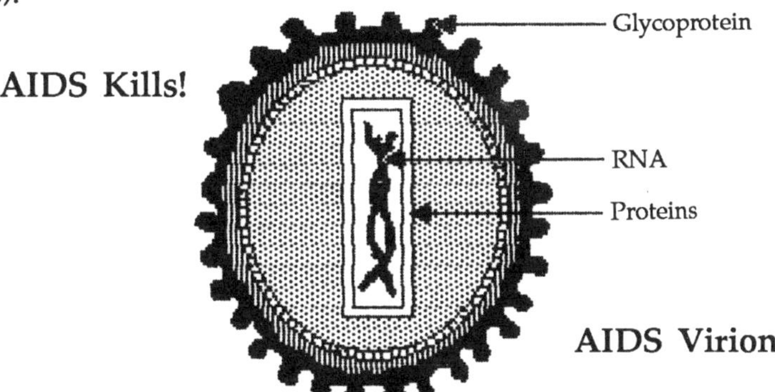

The AIDS virus particle is a sphere that is about 1000 angstroms across. The viral RNA and the enzyme Reverse Transcriptase are carried in the virus's core.

Inside the spherical surface, the core of the AIDS retrovirus contains ribonucleic acid (RNA) along with copies of an enzyme known as "reverse transcriptase" which help the AIDS virion break apart T4-lymphocyte deoxyribonucleic acid (DNA)—the material from which genes, cell reproduction instructions for white blood cells, are made—and assemble and insert its own DNA (viral DNA—genetic machinery) back into the T4-lymphocyte (T4-cell) nucleus. That simple process, assembling and inserting its own DNA into the T4-cell, commandeering the T4-cell genetic machinery to produce more HTLV-III virions, is the first major assault and begins after the HIV retrovirus enters the T4-cell.

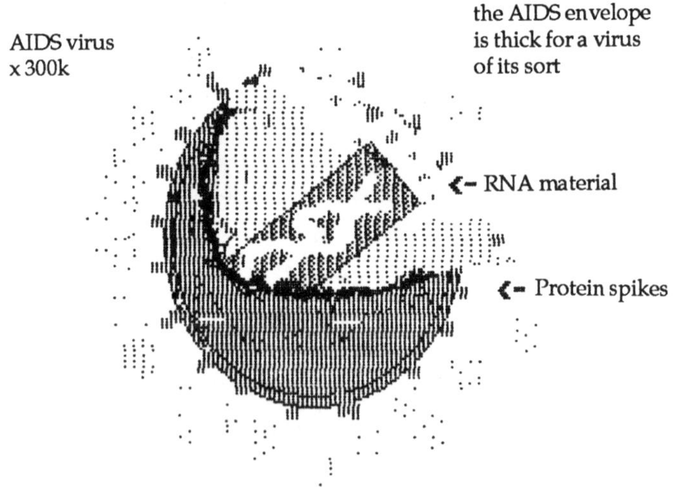

HTLV-III's "immunosuppressive effects in vivo [in a human] are largely paralleled by its ability to selectively infect and kill OKT4 helper/inducer cells in vitro [in the test-tube]"[1] or, simply, the AIDS virion is a highly efficient killer. Dr. William Haseltine of Harvard's Dana-Farber Cancer Institute said in 1985: "Nobody would have thought this level of transcription (production of viral DNA) was possible before . . . It's about 1,000 times faster than the . . . genes we know about."[2] Once HIV is in the T4-cell the battle has been essentially lost. Just how the HIV virion attaches to and penetrates the cell membrane of the T4-cell is a mystery and an area of research in current vaccine development.

The Normal Immunologic Reaction

Why is the embattled T4-cell (white blood cell) so important in fighting disease? The T4-cell is the "trip-wire" of the body's immune system. Prior to a normal microbial or viral infection the T4-cell is in a resting state just waiting for an attack. During infection a cell known as a macrophage (a "disease-scout" cell), after a foreign substance is detected, secretes a protein called 'interleukin-1' (IL-1) and presents an antigen (a protein from the invading organism) to the T4-cell. Once the antigen has been presented to the T4-cell by the macrophage and recognized as foreign, the T4-cell is immunologically activated. Once the T4-cell has been "tripped," many of its genes are turned on—some of which produce interluken-2 (IL-2) and specified receptors (much like a lock awaiting a key) for IL-2.

Once IL-2 (the key), carrying antigens, binds with receptors (lock) located on the T4-cell's surface, the T4-cell, now sensitized to the invading organism's antigens, begins to rapidly reproduce. Each "daughter cell" of the original T4-cell is primed to react to the antigen (foreign body protein) which originally "tripped" the system. These daughter T-4 cells flow through the circulatory (blood) system and, when they encounter an antigen to which they have been programmed to respond, trigger the maturation of B-lymphocytes and T8-leukocytes (T8-cells) in that immediate area. Both the mature B-lymphocytes (through produced antibodies) and T8-cells then directly attack the invader.

The Immune System and AIDS

In war, surprise attack is a cherished strategy. Better yet is the conversion of the palace guard to the side of the enemy —treason kills the king. Such is the strategy of the AIDS virion: a very finely tuned biomolecular treason. First, HTLV-III targets any T4-molecule-bearing macrophages (those disease-scout cells originally designed to present antigens to the T4-cells). Thus a "scout," being made "treasonous," may carry the very enemy (AIDS) to the "tripwire." Second, through some as yet unknown method(s), HTLV-III enters the T4-cell before a sufficient immune system response can be developed and, stealthily, HIV begins causing genetic changes within the T4-cell's DNA material. Finally, to complete the mutiny, infected T4-cells may lie "dormant" (although genetically mutated) until an immunologic response is triggered by another foreign antigen, perhaps by a cytomegalovirus attack.

When an immunological reaction is provoked through presentation of antigens from other foreign invaders, the treasonous T4-cell displays its true colors. The IL-2 receptor reaction occurs as expected but, rather than producing hundreds of sensitized daughters, only a few (often less than 20) daughters are produced. Further, instead of the expected stimulation to maturity of B-lymphocytes and T8-cells to directly confront the new (non-HTLV-III) invader, thousands of HIV virions are produced in the few remaining daughters by the commandeered DNA. HTLV-III "produces a trans-activating protein that greatly stimulates the expression of viral genes. In that regard, it resembles HTLV-I and -II which cause human leukemias or lymphomas."[3]

However, the treasonous T4-cell daughters are short-lived, their death coming in the explosive birthing of more AIDS virions—an event which literally tears the T4-cell to shreds. As AIDS progresses, the T-4 cell population dwindles, B-lymphocytes and T8-cells fail to mature, and any foreign invader is free to roam and multiply—the immune system has been "decapitated." With each bout of an opportunistic infection, the remaining commandeered T4-cells contribute more HTLV-III virions further suppressing any remaining potential of the host for fighting any disease. The infected person has acquired an immune deficiency, a form of "contagious cancer" gradually killing the body's normal T4 (white) blood cells.

AIDS and the Infected Individual

In those persons infected with AIDS, a continuing progression of diseases begins which often leads to the initial diagnosis of AIDS. Among those opportunistic diseases frequently seen in AIDS victims are:

1. *Pneumocystis carinii,* a lung infection caused by protozoa
2. *Kaposi's sarcoma,* an especially virulent form of skin cancer

3. *Candidiasis,* a fungal condition that in AIDS patients commonly affects the mouth and esophagus
4. *Cytomegalovirus,* a viral infection which can lead to meningitis and colitis
5. A host of atypical bacterial infections, many of which attack the liver or bone marrow
6. Chronic *Herpes Zoster,* an ulceration of either the oral or anal area
7. *Cryptosporidiosis,* an organism causing prolonged diarrhea
8. *Toxoplasmosis,* a protozoan infection which targets the brain and eyes

The progression of disease continues until death—no one has been known to recover from AIDS. As of March 1987, this battle had been waged and lost by over 19,000 Americans.

Where did AIDS come from?

The countries of the world showing the highest rates of infection are located in south-central Africa. Epidemiological studies have confirmed that HTLV-III spread first in Africa and is endemic in Zaire, Burundi, Uganda, Rwanda, Tanzania, and Kenya. "Tests on (blood) sera from the 1960's and 1970's detect no antibodies to HTLV-III anywhere except in a small region of central Africa, where the earliest signs of infection have been found in serum samples taken in the 1950's."[4] Time regression of AIDS growth suggests the possibility of its origin in the early 1940's (1941). Location regression of AIDS spread suggests the possibility of its origin in, or very near, eastern Zaire, near the northern tip of Lake Tanganyika.

The actual genesis of the AIDS virus has not been discovered, yet many unusual ideas and/or rumors have been advanced by sundry persons and organizations. It has been observed that uranium and radium mining and smelting occurred in the southeastern Zaire region (formerly the Shinkolobwe Mine, operated by Union Miniere, near Jadotville, which was 87 miles northwest of Elisabethville in the Belgium Congo), which supplied fission material for U.S. nuclear weapons until approximately 1955. Prevailing winds in that area are from the southwest. It is argued that perhaps escaped radiation from uranium smelting provoked a genetic mutation in a virus. Reports from the Lyndon LaRouche organization have stated that AIDS and other lethal contagions were "deliberately created by the International Monetary Fund, that Henry Kissinger and Zionism somehow played a role by curtailing U.S. biological warfare abilities and helped open the door to AIDS, and that U.S. policy on AIDS is dictated by the Soviet government via the World Health Organization."[5] Still others have credited the genesis of AIDS to either American or Soviet biological warfare experiments gone awry as well as extraterrestrial origin from within stony meteorites.

Probably none of these "rumors" are accurate—the scientific community generally supports the notion that the genesis of AIDS was a result of a naturally occurring genetic mutation of a formerly harmless retrovirus. Hopefully, clearer heads will prevail regarding AIDS genesis. None of these "rumors" is conducive to logical interpretation of the epidemic or helpful in meeting the problems at hand.

AIDS in Africa

"In Africa, as many as 2 million to 5 million may already be infected and in ten years," predicts Epidemiologist B. Frank Polk of Johns Hopkins University, "some countries could lose 25% of their population. The [African] loss in terms of the economy and social structure could well equal the black death's ruination of medieval Europe."[6] David Baltimore says "[AIDS] threatens to undermine countries, particularly in [central] Africa. It will cause such a significant amount of disease in the middle ages of the population that it will largely reduce the number of people available to carry out the functions of the society. In parts of [that continent], it's happening now."

"In the epicenter" (Uganda and Zaire), says Belgian Microbiologist Peter Piot, "15% to 25% of the adult population is affected [with AIDS]."[8] Dr. Samuel Okware, the Ministry of Health official in charge of Uganda's AIDS prevention program has stated: "In the year 2000, one in every two sexually active adults will be infected."[9] *Atlantic Monthly* reported the following comment made on National Public Radio: "The World Health Organization has written off—completely written off—four central African countries because the level of AIDS infection is so high."[10] Dr. Cranmer Terrace, Department of Clinical Pharmacology at St. George's Hospital Medical School in London, stated: "Developed countries cannot stand by and allow AIDS to devastate and . . . destabilize central Africa, and later . . . South America and possibly [other areas]."[11] The inference appears clear—these countries may, without unparalleled intervention, simply cease to exist.

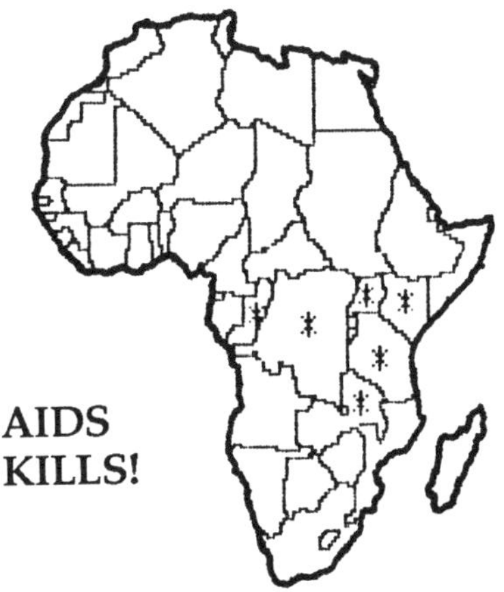

Africa
The AIDS retrovirus began as a mutation of an apparently harmless retrovirus found in the African Green Monkey during the 1940's or 1950's. AIDS has been found in high incidence in Zaire, Burundi, Uganda, Rwanda, Tanzania, and Kenya.

The Advent of AIDS in Humankind

In Africa, the Green Monkey (Cercopithecus aethiops) may have been a first link to human AIDS infection. That primate carries a virus (Simian T-lymphotropic virus, or STLV-III) that is similar to the HTLV-III AIDS virus. Although STLV-III does not cause illness in the Green monkey, scientists at the New England Primate Center in Southborough, Massachusetts noticed that STLV-III was fatal to rhesus macaque monkeys. Virologists Max Essex and Phyllis Kanki, both of Harvard University, found one-half to two-thirds of Green Monkeys in the African AIDS belt to be infected with the simian equivalent of HTLV-III. The animals are known to forage in garbage dumps and, when people try to chase them away, sometimes fight back by biting and scratching. Additionally, Africans in the Burundi/Zaire area are fond of eating monkeys—a practice through which humans may have come into contact with the STLV-III virus. Such close contact with infected animals, some scientists think, was how the virus found its way into humans.

Other scientists have discovered apparently intermediate viruses (HTLV-IV, Lymphoadenopathy Virus-2 [LAV-2], SBL virus) between STLV-III and HTLV-III in West Africa suggesting "that somehow STLV-III entered humans and initiated a series of mutations that yielded the intermediate viruses before finally terminating in the fierce pathology of HTLV-III."[12] "It is therefore conceivable that STLV-III or HTLV-IV (another AIDS-related virus) may have served as the progenitor virus to the human AIDS virus; alternatively they (the retrovirus group) may have had a common progenitor"[13] not yet discovered.

Where has AIDS Spread?

About 113 nations have reported cases of AIDS, but information from many countries may be unreliable due to the newness of the disease and the lack of expertise in many of the Third-World national health systems in either diagnosis or record-keeping. Those nations with more reliable data as of January 1987 showed cases of AIDS by country: Zambia: an estimated 15% of its 6 million population may be infected (900,000); the United States: 32,000; Brazil: 1,110; France: 806; West Germany: 675; Britain: 548; Switzerland: 170; Japan: 21; and, the Soviet Union: 12.

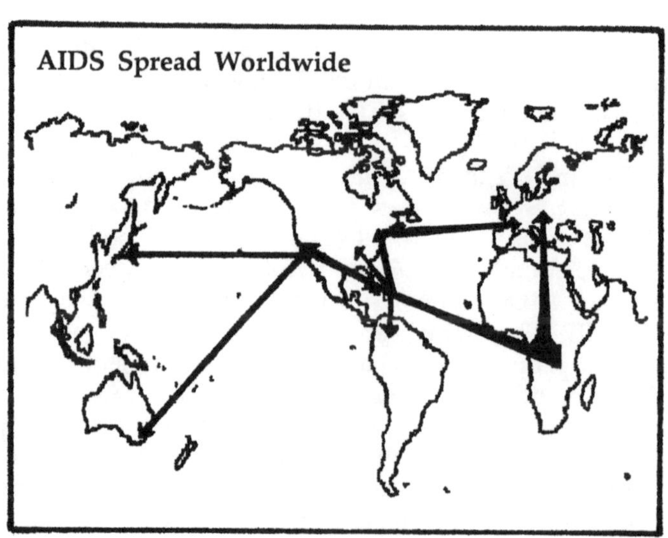

"It appears that after remaining localized for some time [in Africa], the virus began spreading to the rest of central Africa during the early 1970's. Later in that decade it reached Haiti and may have reached Europe and the Americas from there."[14] As of March 1987, AIDS had spread to nearly every nation of the earth. So far 39% of AIDS cases in the U.S. have been in New York and San Francisco. Recent data shows "One in 50 people in Manhattan between the ages of 18 and 25 who apply for military service are infected by the AIDS virus."[15]

Who is at Risk for AIDS?

At first (1981) AIDS seemed to be a disease strictly of the homosexual male community. However, as time passed several high-risk groups seemed to emerge. These identified high-risk groups by type and number infected as of October 1986 were:

Risk Group	Number	% of All Cases
Homosexual and bisexual men*	18,587	72.5%
Intravenous drug users	4,322	16.8%
Hemophiliacs	215	.8%
Transfusion recipients	436	1.7%
Children	354	1.4%
Heterosexuals	959	3.7%
No known risk factors	777	3.0%
Total	25,650	

*Includes 4322 who are also intravenous drug users.[16]

Of the more than 29,000 U.S. cases, 73 percent have been homosexual or bisexual men (including homosexual intravenous drug abusers), 17 percent intravenous drug users (non-homosexual), 4 percent heterosexuals and 3 percent persons who received blood or blood products (a third of whom have been people with hemophilia or other blood disorders). While it is true that male homosexuals and bisexuals account for about 75 percent of AIDS cases, percentages of distribution of the disease are changing.

There have been about 450 cases in children. However, "the syndrome is apparently not transmitted through casual household contact and hence not among school children."[17]

Other research appears to indicate that AIDS is not selective of any group and is spreading to the general population. Dr. Robert Redfield has pointed out that studies of 1970's frozen blood sera of the gay San Francisco population showed 1 in every 1000 cases seropositive, but, "Today, one in a thousand such samples are infected in the *general* population," suggesting grave concern about AIDS's spread.[18]

Dr. Robert Gallo, a noted authority on AIDS in the United States, reported "Analysis of the origin and spread of HTLV-III leads to a conclusion that cannot be sufficiently emphasized: AIDS is not a disease of homosexuals or drug addicts or indeed of any particular risk group." He continued, "The virus is spread by intimate contact, and the form of contact seems to be less important than the contact itself. Rapid spread of the virus depends on the accumulation of a pool of infected people that is large enough for a few exposures to result in infection. The pool need not consist of homosexuals or drug addicts. In Africa, the pool is made up of heterosexuals, and others have demonstrated heterosexual transmission in the U.S."[19] In other words, Gallo is saying that as more persons become infected, the greater the risk may be to those who are not.

"Heterosexual transmission, at least in Haiti and Africa, is becoming increasingly prevalent . . . and the virus may have been around as long ago as 1962."[20] Mid-1987 data suggests that approximately 7 percent of AIDS cases now exist in the heterosexual population. By 1991 (in the United States), according to the most conservative estimates, 270,000 people will have been stricken, 179,000 will have died—and new cases involving heterosexuals will have multiplied 10-fold to 23,000 (and that is a low estimate). Almost 4,000 babies will have contracted AIDS. The Centers for Disease Control (CDC) in Atlanta estimates that 50,000 persons may die of AIDS in 1991 alone—as many as die annually in traffic accidents. Concern exists among some scientists that the situation in Africa, where men and women are equally infected, may foreshadow what is to come in the United States.

As of March 1987, the AIDS epidemic was still highly concentrated among two groups, homosexual/bisexual males and intravenous drug abusers—but this may not, as time passes, continue. "Their" disease has suddenly and will continue to become "our" disease.

What Spreads AIDS from Person to Person?

"The rectum, the lower portion of the large intestine that ends in the anus, is lined with fragile, easily [injured] columnar cells. Moreover, the closer to the anus, the more blood vessels there are [and the more likely a blood-letting injury]. Anal intercourse, second only to oral sex in frequency among homosexuals, can tear the lining [of the rectum] allowing AIDS virus-infected semen ready entry to the blood stream."[21] Additionally, the lining of the male urethra, the narrow tube leading from the bladder to the penis through which urine is evacuated, is also lined with these same easily injured cells and numerous underlying blood vessels.

During anal intercourse with an AIDS-infected partner, the AIDS virus can easily pass from the rectum into the urethra or vice versa, where the virus can easily penetrate any injury in the fragile lining and enter into the blood stream. The practice of frequent anal intercourse and "fisting" (insertion of the hand into a sex partner's rectum), both of which may cause bleeding in the rectum, can transmit the infection. Any sexual behavior in which blood/body fluid exchange is possible can, potentially, be responsible for transfection of another individual: anal intercourse, oral-genital sex, oral-anal sex, or other acts through which body fluids may be transferred.

Consider the following chart of risk behavior:

Correlation Direction	Activity	R^2	P
positive	Number of Partners	4.49	.03
positive	Receptive Anal Intercourse	4.91	.03
negative	Insertive Anal Intercourse	6.62	.01
negative	Receptive Fisting	.16	.70
positive	Insertive Fisting	4.06	.04
positive	Receptive Analingus	2.35	.10
negative	Insertive Analingus	1.74	.20
negative	Receptive Fellatio	.42	.50
negative	Insertive Fellatio	2.36	.10
positive	Nitrite Inhalant Frequency	1.33	.20
positive	Number of Partners and Receptive Anal Intercourse	8.71	.003 [22]

The above data shows a number of homosexual behaviors increasing risk. The most dangerous condition is receptive anal intercourse with a large number of different individuals, with a chance of only 3 in 1000 that it does *not* spread AIDS.

The AIDS virus has also been found in breast milk and vaginal secretions making both breast feeding and heterosexual intercourse potential transmission behaviors. As of March 1987, several U.S. cities have reported, in random samples of prostitutes, an AIDS-infection rate rising over 30%. Newly published studies on male and female AIDS patients and their partners indicate that the disease is bi-directional, that is, transmissible equally easily by both men and women. In central Africa, incidence among prostitutes is much higher than in the United States; e.g., "27% in Zaire carry AIDS virus antibodies, 59% in Kenya, and 88% in Rwanda,"[23] but this is likely to change as the percentage of infected American prostitutes increases. "Some [American] studies indicate that a woman who has frequent sex with a carrier of the virus has a 33%-50% chance of becoming infected—roughly the same as for catching syphilis or gonorrhea.[24] A six-month study in Alameda County, California found the number of women showing a positive test for AIDS antibodies was "the same percentage reported in women who came to county clinics for treatment of syphilis, gonorrhea or other sexual diseases."[25]

Heterosexuals have been warned of "safe sex" practices —avoiding fellatio, vaginal and anal sex without a condom, and cunnilingus without a shield. Researchers often recommend using latex condoms and diaphragms, in adjunct with a water-soluble lubricant containing 5% nonoxynol-9, as a way to reduce the risk of transmission. However, because of other information about potential transfection soon to be presented, caution is advised. Survey data in the United States, including a military study, and on the tremendous spread of the disease in Africa, indicate that AIDS is passed as easily from women to men as from men to their sexual partners. Research conducted by Dr. Robert Redfield shows 50% of the spouses of infected partners contract AIDS, regardless of whether the spouse was male or female. The transmission of AIDS is typical of other sexually transmitted diseases: deep-kissing, sexual intercourse and, particularly, sexual practices involving the rectal mucosa, are dangerous and may lead to disease transmission. Blood transfusions, organ transplantation, and artificial insemination can also spread AIDS, albeit, the risk from blood transfusion appears slight. The reader is advised, however, that in some cases donors with AIDS may *never* show seropositive HIV antibodies, and autologous blood transfusions are the only means of absolutely insuring no risk.

To summarize information available as of March 1987, any sexual behavior through which body fluids (semen, urine, saliva, blood, feces, sweat, lymph, breast milk, vaginal secretions, and tears) are exchanged, and particularly come into contact with either yours or another's blood (small cuts in rectum, urethra, vagina, mouth/gums, fingers; other open wounds, abrasions, or blemishes) only ONCE is potentially sufficient to spread the disease. Multiple exposures to the virus are apparently not required for heterosexual transmission. A study by the Centers for Disease Control found a case of a woman who tested sero-positive for AIDS after only one sexual encounter with her husband who, through transfusion, had contracted the disease. As previously mentioned, use of condoms has been advocated as a means to reduce the spread of the disease, but condoms must be used carefully; during withdrawal, hold the base of the condom tightly around the penis so that the condom cannot slip off and no semen can escape. Further, condoms must be latex rubber—because of the size of the HIV virion, animal skin condoms appear likely to allow the retrovirus passage through the condom membrane.

More Concerns About AIDS Spread

The potential spread of AIDS can be grasped by observing the ways in which other sexually transmitted diseases, such as gonorrhea, chlamydia, and genital herpes, move through the country. "There are a minimum of 6 million S.T.D.'s recorded annually," says Dr. German Maisonet, medical director of the Los Angeles Minority AIDS Project, "which means that about every five seconds an American is involved in a high-risk sexual practice minus a condom." Other behaviors of suspicion include tatooing, and blood-to-blood contact—such as a wrist-to-wrist blood-brother/sister exchange. "Children may not have sexual relations with one another, the commonest way to pass on AIDS, but they fight, have nose bleeds and play at being "blood brothers" by mixing their blood."[27] How many children have cuts and scratches?

Certainly, one sure method of assuring minimal risk of exposure without use of "safe sex" procedures is remaining celebate. Another is maintaining a sexual relationship—in which neither partner abuses intravenous drugs—which has been exclusively monogamous for approximately 15 years during which time no blood transfusions were received. When beginning a new monogamous sexual relationship, the partners should rely upon strict celebacy and continued quarterly (every 3 months) sero-negative reports (test reports showing absence of AIDS anti-bodies in the blood) for a period of one year before commencing any sexual activity. In any case where monogamy has not occurred or a sexual relationship is newer than 15 years of age, a degree of risk exists.

Any cut, lesion, abrasion, or blemish in the presence of the AIDS virion may, potentially, lead to disease spread. Three health care workers were reported by the CDC to have contracted AIDS following non-needle-stick exposures to blood from infected patients. Worker 1 "may have had a small amount of infected blood on her index finger for about 20 minutes before washing her hands. She had no open wounds, but her hands were chapped." Worker 2 had infected blood spattered "on her face and in her mouth . . . She had facial acne but no open wounds. She washed the blood off immediately after the exposure." Worker 3 had infected blood "covering most of her hands and forearms. She was not wearing gloves. She does not recall having any open wounds on her hands or any mucous-membrane exposure. However, she had dermatitis on one ear and may have touched it."[28] To assure minimum risk of infection, all breaks in the skin should be covered and contact with mucous-membranes should be prevented.

Additionally, some medical procedures may inadvertently contribute to the spread of the disease. J. A. Clarke, of Queen Mary's Hospital, London, reported a case where a skin allograft (a temporary skin transplant) "used as a temporary wound dressing was taken from a patient who later proved to have antibodies to HIV [and] . . . the skin was used before the serological results [of HIV status] was available." The receiving patient subsequently tested seropositive for HIV. He concludes, "The transfer of HIV in a skin graft should pre-empt re-evaluation of the long-established practice of using sheets of allograft until autograft cover can be achieved" or, simply, don't use a skin graft except as a last resort.[29] Further, in another medically related incident, it was reported at the Third Annual International Conference on AIDS in Washington, D.C. (May 31-June 5, 1987) that a dentist in the state of New York had apparently contracted AIDS from one of his patients, and the probable means of transfection was through saliva contact with an open sore on his hand. How many additional dental patients were served by this dentist after his infection and before he was aware of his condition and what risk is therein associated for these patients?

Insect Vectors?

Researchers Mark Whiteside and Caroline MacLeod, of the Institute of Tropical Medicine, Miami, Florida, have proposed that insects, particularly mosquitoes, may play a role in spreading AIDS, although Harold Jaffee, deputy director of the AIDS task force of the Centers for Disease Control, states, "We know the AIDS virus is unusually picky in the kinds of cells it chooses to live in so it's very unlikely that it could live in insect cells, which are very different from human cells in morphology and function."[30]

Other more recent research compounds the debate. Researchers of the Pasteur Institute (Paris, France) have shown that in Zaire, "the presence of DNA sequences homologous to the HIV virus in the genome of insects (tse tse flies, fruit flies, cockroaches, antlions, ticks) captured in Zaire or in the Central African Republic, a zone endemic of the virus, reinforces the idea of the possibility of the transmission of AIDS in this way and of the formation of a natural reservoir for the virus. . . ."[31] A. Srinivasan, of the Retrovirus Diseases Branch of the CDC in Atlanta, reported: "The lack of HIV replication and HIV-LTR-directed CAT expression in arthropod cells may be due to ineffectiveness of the HIV promoter and not to lack of entry of DNA which was shown by DNA-uptake experiments."[32] In simple terms, the AIDS virus can invade the genetic material of insects but does not replicate while in insects because a growth promoter is absent.

Dr. Thomas Quinn, from the National Institute of Allergy and Infectious Diseases in Bethesda, Maryland, through epidemiological research in Africa, found that sex, not mosquitoes, was mainly responsible for the spread of AIDS. "It is possible that a mosquito could fly from one person to another with blood on its proboscis (stinger) and take the virus with it. Bed bugs may spread hepatitis B this way. But mosquitoes would do this only when interrupted in mid-course".[33] However, there appears a possibility. Dr. Robert C. Gallo recently (March 1987) cited epidemiologically sound data from London and Trinidad where HTLV-I, a retrovirus associated with leukemia and similar in structure to AIDS, can be transmitted by the household mosquito.

An article in *The Lancet* (July 5, 1986) poses the possibility that mechanical transmission of HIV between persons could be carried out by bedbugs. Similar to the previous discussion regarding possibilities for transmission by mosquitoes, Lyons states, "Mechanical transmission depends upon an insect being interrupted while feeding on an infected host and then moving to a susceptible host to complete its blood meal. Transmission would occur via contaminated mouthparts and/or regurgitation,"[34] particularly possible in the bedbugs *Rhodnius prolixus* and possibly in *Cimex lectularius*. Lyon's team found that HIV could exist for 1 hour in *Cimex lectularius* following a feeding on infected blood. It appears involvement of insects in the spread of AIDS remains controversial (as of March 1987), while research continues.

Food Preparation as a Vector?

Whether the HTLV-III virus can be transmitted through food or drink products has not been demonstrated. AIDS thrives in a 'chilly' environment, and heat de-activates it easily. If a sample suspended in a fluid-filled test-tube is left to stand at room temperature for 24 hours, it has only a ten per cent chance of surviving. Other research has shown that the AIDS virus can be inactivated by high and low pH and by exposure to a temperature of 56 degrees Celcius (about 100 degrees Farenheit) for 10 minutes. Still other research cited on pp. 721-22 in the September 28, 1985 issue of *The Lancet* indicates the AIDS virus can *live at room temperature for as long as 10 days even if dried.* These data seem to suggest that the virus can survive in an ambient (normal room-temperature) environment for a relatively long period, but heat can easily kill the virus. T4-cells and macrophages, which the AIDS virus favors, are "not usually found in the upper digestive tract, a fact that makes food a highly unlikely[35] but not totally discounted transmitter.

Common household cleaners and detergents, including bleach and even hand soap, will kill the virus. It is an apparent possibility, albeit exceedingly small, that AIDS could be spread through unsanitary preparation of non-cooked food (e.g., body fluid from an infected person contacts a non-cooked food; another person with mouth/gum lesions ingests that food allowing the virus entry into the blood). Further research is needed and that research needs to be made public.

Possibilities of Casual Contact?

Michael Gottlieb, a UCLA Medical Center immunologist, in 1985 stated, "There's absolutely no evidence that it can be spread by a cough or a sneeze or by shaking hands with a person with the disease who has *no* open sores."[36] This observation by Gottlieb is interesting when compared to nursing protocol with coughing or sneezing AIDS patients: wear a mask and goggles when you perform procedures that might involve flying droplets of body fluid from an AIDS patient or fluid from aerosols. As the AIDS virion is found in saliva and T4 macrophages (the original target of the HIV) are found in the lungs, then it appears a possibility of transfection from coughing or sneezing. Again, specific research needs to be conducted and that research needs to be made public.

According to *U.S. News and World Report,* "no known cases have been transmitted [through shaking hands, hugging, social kissing, crying, coughing, sneezing, French Kissing, eating food prepared by someone with AIDS, or insect bites]."[37] Of apparent possible contradiction and certainly a poignant observation, Barbara Amiel, writing in *Maclean's,* said, "I saw medical staff [involved in AIDS-related work] all bundled up like mummies [in research laboratories and hospitals]. As far as I could see, the medical staff were not going to have sex with AIDS patients nor were they taking blood transfusions, but their protective clothing far exceeded the normal masks and gowns one might expect in a hospital. They were clearly worried about tears, sweat and saliva."[38]

From a strictly scientific viewpoint, testing any of these possibilities can only be done with chimpanzees and, despite an exhaustive search, this writer has located no information which scientifically proves or disproves these possibilities. Information concerning health practitioner care precautions with AIDS victims provokes a degree of suspicion concerning the AIDS transfection as expressed by Amiel. Dr. Robert Gallo, in March

1987, said regarding casual contact as a factor for AIDS spread, "I think it's remote since the virus would have to change so much, but we just don't know if it will happen." He went on to say that he could not rule out the possibility of casual contact spreading the disease some time in the future if the virus mutates greatly.[39] Perhaps there is need for concern—at least for definitive scientific study?

Health Care Provider Precautions

Health-care practitioners who work with AIDS infected individuals in either a home or hospital setting are instructed that they should give special attention to good handwashing techniques. If the health-care attendant has open cuts or sores on the hands, gloves should be worn when dealing with the infected individual. The health-care attendant should always wear gloves when direct contact with the patient's body fluids such as blood, sputum, feces, urine, saliva, vomitus or semen is possible. Solid health-care related wastes such as tissues, gloves and disposable items, which come in contact with body fluids, should be disposed of in securely tied double plastic bags.

All eating and food preparation utensils should be washed thoroughly with hot water and liquid soap—the health-care attendant wearing dishwashing gloves to protect chapping of the hands (and opening of wounds). If the health-care attendant is attending an infected person whose body fluids will come in contact with the health-care attendant's clothing, a smock or apron should be worn—the apron and all soiled clothing and linen should be washed frequently with detergent and a 1% chlorine bleach. For visitors to an AIDS-infected person's home, gloves, gowns and mask are utilized if visitors will be in contact with body fluids or if visitors have contagious conditions.

If the infected person is coughing, sneezing, or producing sputum, the health-care attendant should keep disposable tissues within that person's reach, along with a receptacle for the soiled tissues. Further, the health-care attendant is advised to encourage the patient to cover his mouth when sneezing or coughing.

In-Home Family Health Care Precautions

Advice for a family treating an AIDS-infected person at home is equally important. "The patient's razor, toothbrush, and personal hygiene items that might come in contact with his body secretions must be his *alone.* The same is true for his washcloths and towels between launderings. Before giving care, check your hands. If you see any cuts, wear gloves. If exposed to diarrheic or bloody secretions, wear gloves. Should you accidentally touch or be splashed by these secretions, wash the explosed area with hydrogen peroxide.

The patient's soiled linen does not belong in the household hamper. Keep it in plastic bags until it's ready to be laundered. Do not overload the washing machine to allow detergent to circulate freely; use detergent and a phenolic disinfectant (such as Lysol); use a second wash to remove any remaining chemicals.

After spills (such as body secretions or bath water) are cleaned up with soap and water, the area should be wiped with a solution of bleach and water at a ratio of 1:10; full-strength bleach is best for cleaning the toilet bowl. Dirty water from cleaning the bathroom (or body secretion spills) should be flushed down the toilet and mops and sponges soaked for 5 minutes in the 1:10 bleach-water solution. However, they should be used for cleaning the bathroom only, not for general household cleaning. Similarly, another set should be kept aside for cleaning body secretion spills in other parts of the house. All the family's kitchen utensils and dishes can be washed together in *hot* soapy water and air dried."[40]

Whether the extremely active effort toward maintaining a "germ-free" environment is based upon the needs of the immunologically-deprived AIDS person or the health of the family is not important; the likely requirement is for protection of both parties. Certainly the continued exposure of the family and/or health-care attendant would appear to increase the degree of risk of transfection, and, because of the advice given to both family and health-care attendants alike, there appears to be a need for further public assurance regarding the inability of casual contact to cause transfection. It is widely stated that AIDS is hard to contract, barring high-risk group behavior, yet concern continues among the general public as a result of lack of solid empirical scientific data. Correlational studies and the opinion of experts does not appear to be sufficiently convincing to allay public concern—nor, by the way, is it good science.

A study conducted by Dr. Gerald Friedman at Montefiore Hospital in New York showed that "despite prolonged and close contact with patients who have AIDS or ARC, one hundred of one-hundred-and-one household contacts did not catch infection."[41] One person did—how? Dr. Wade Parks of the University of Miami (Florida) found, in 45 persons married to AIDS patients, that 65% of the men and 54% of the women non-infected spouses eventually contracted the virus, but not through non-sexual casual contact. Were scientific controls used to assure the validity of his conclusions? Whether, in fact, the disease is spread through casual contact must be scientifically proven through controlled laboratory animal research or through strictly controlled experimentation with couples where one member is infected before nonequivocal statements can be made. Again, correlational research and insufficient scientifically-controlled observation does not demonstrate cause and effect. To this writer's knowledge, these experiments have not yet been conducted or have not been sufficiently publicized. If research regarding casual contact potential has not been sufficiently publicized, a knowledgable person must question why.

AIDS Transmission and the School Environment

The controversy provoked by school-age, AIDS-infected children attending classes suggests the need for exact experimentation and public education of the results of those cases. The American Academy of Pediatrics and the CDC recommend most school-age children and adolescents with AIDS attend school with the approval of their physician. Yet, also recommended are restrictive educational environments for younger children: the neurologically handicapped, the incontinent, or aggressive biting children, suggesting, in some cases, casual contact may be of concern as a result of childrens' indiscriminate contact with body fluids. A study by Dr. Jerome Groopman of Harvard University, reported a case where an elderly man, infected by AIDS through transfusion, *did* infect his wife through *only* kissing.

A case of horizontal transmission (i.e., apparent casual contact) between two siblings was reported in the September 20, 1986 issue of *The Lancet*. Observed in Germany, a HIV-seropositive three and a half year-old child died from AIDS and later his six and a half year-old brother became ill with the disease. It was reported that the older brother "had never been seriously ill, had never been given blood or blood products, and had not been sexually abused" and neither were there bedbugs in the home nor were any other members of the family infected with the retrovirus. Wahn stated, "One possible route of virus transmission was a bite on the older brother's forearm by the younger child about 6 months before he died. The mother had seen teeth imprints on the skin but no bleeding or haematoma. This observation suggests that even minor bites by HIV infected children may carry the risk of virus transmission."[42]

In a study to determine the transmissibility of HIV between hemophilic and non-hemophilic children in a private school setting in France, A. Berthier reported, "half of the hemophilic children had seroconverted (became HIV-infected) by the end of a 3-year study period. By contrast, none of the nonhemophilic children seroconverted." However, it was reported that "Hepatitis B virus (HBV) markers detected in all poly-transfused hemophiliacs were found in 4 of 20 control children in the school, whereas all healthy youngsters living with their families were HBV negative."[43] Of potential concern, other experts in the field have remarked that the transmissibility of HBV is very similar to that of AIDS. Could a longer period of "close contact" have resulted in transmission?

John R. Seale, formerly a consultant venereologist (specialist in venereal diseases) of the Middlesex and St. Thomas Hospitals in London, England, said, "With infected cells and virions intermittently shed in saliva, semen and vaginal secretions, and several million people already infected, transmission during biologically normal sexual intercourse is beginning to escalate. *Furthermore, now that large numbers of children have been infected, transmission between infants and young children via infectious blood and saliva is inevitable.* [emphasis added][44] Clearly, less litigation and "expert opinion" and more exact scientific experimentation is necessary to develop an educated, prepared public.

Epilogue

The head of the United Nations' World Health Organization, Halfdan Mahler, has remarked that AIDS "is a health disaster of pandemic proportions" and the National Academy of Sciences has criticized the U.S. Government effort to attack the AIDS pandemic as "woefully inadequate."[45] "Without decisive action," Institute of Medicine president Samuel Thier says, "the epidemic may snowball into an even greater catastrophe"[46] and the "potential damage done to modern society by AIDS would compare with that expected from a nuclear war between the major powers,"[47] but relatively little in terms of federal government or public health leadership to avert such a catastrophe has yet surfaced.

At the present AIDS growth, by the year 2001 (14 years from this writing), the United States may potentially—that year alone—show 3.5 million diagnosed, 50 million infected but not yet diagnosed, and 1.5 million dying. Over 20% of the U.S. population could be involved in the pandemic, of which most would be between 20 and 60 years old (nearly 30 million persons). If a vaccine does not appear until the turn of the century, the death toll could be in the tens of millions, and so far AIDS shows no sign of dying out on its own.

Dr. David Stevens, chief of infectious diseases at Santa Clara County Valley Medical Center, said during January 1987, "The numbers are staggering. We have a megaproblem approaching us in this county [indeed in the nation] and I don't think that fact has been grasped by many people."[48] America is not, but must be, prepared for this.

Notes

[1]Fisher, A. G., et al. "Infectious Mutants of HTLV-III with Changes in the 3' Region and Markedly Reduced Cytopathic Effects," *Science* 233.4764: 65.

[2]Antonio, G. THE AIDS COVER-UP? (San Francisco: Ignatius Press, 1987) 6.

[3]Marx, J. L. "A Surprising Action for the AIDS Virus," *Science* 231. 4740: 798.

[4]Gallo, R. C. "The AIDS Virus," *Scientific American* 256.1: 56.

[5]Petit, C. "California to Vote on AIDS Proposition," *Science* 234.4774: 278.

[6]Wallis, C. "You Haven't Heard Anything Yet," *Time*, Feb. 16, 1987: 54.

[7]"Quarantining Will Help No One," an interview with AIDS expert and Nobel laureate David Baltimore, *U. S. News and World Report*, Jan. 12, 1987: 70.

[8]Serrill, Michael S. "In the Grip of the Scourge," *Time*, Feb. 16, 1987: 59.

[9]Serrill 58.

[10]Leishman, K. "Heterosexuals and AIDS," *Atlantic Monthly*, Feb. 1987: 44.

[11]Terrace, C. "AIDS in Africa," *Nature*, Vol. 232: 104.

[12]Gallo 56.

[13]Kanki, P. J., et al. "New Human T-Lymphotropic Retrovirus Related to Simian T-Lymphotropic Virus Type III (STLV-III AGM)," *Science* 232.4747: 243.

[14]Gallo 56.

[15]Barnes, D. M. "Military Statistics on AIDS in the U.S.," *Science* 233. 4761: 283.

[16]Norman, C. "Sex and Needles, Not Insects and Pigs, Spread AIDS in Florida Town," *Science* 234.4775: 416.

[17]Silberner, J. "AIDS: Casual Contact Exonerated," *Science News* 128. 14: 213.

[18]Fettner, A. "Women and AIDS," *Health*, Nov. 1986: 62.

[19]Gallo 56.

[20]Silberner 213.

[21]Lagone, J. "AIDS: Special Report." *Discover* 6.12: 40.

[22]Devita, Jr., M.D. "*AIDS: Etiology, Diagnosis, Treatment and Prevention* (Philadelphia: 1985) 16-17.

[23]Barnes, D. M. "Unsuspected Prevalence of AIDS in Africa"; *Science* 233.476: 282.

[24]Hamilton, J. O., et al. "The AIDS Epidemic and Business," *Business Week*, March 23, 1987: 130.

[25]Cohn, A. "Doctor Conducted Secret AIDS Tests," *San Jose (California) Mercury News*, Jan. 21, 1987.

[26]Smilgis, Martha. "The Big Chill: Fear of AIDS," *Time*, Feb.16, 1987: 53.

[27]Amiel, B. "The Politics of a Killer Disease," *Maclean's*, Dec. 8, 1986: 11.

[28]"Update: Human Immunodeficiency Virus Infections in Health-Care Workers Exposed to Blood of Infected Patients," *Morbidity and Mortality Weekly Report* 36.19: 285-86.

[29]Clarke, J. A. "HIV Transmission and Skin Grafts," *The Lancet*, April 25, 1987: 983.

[30]"A Dissenter in the AIDS Capital of the World," *Discover* Dec. 1985: 48.

[31]Becker, J.-L., et al. "Infection de cellules d'insectes en culture par le virus HIV, agent du SIDA, et mise en 'evidence d'insectes d'origine africaine contamine's par ce virus," *Acade'mie des Sciences*, t. 303, S'rie III, no. 8: 306.

[32]Srinivasan, A., et al. "Lack of HIV Replication in Arthropod Cells," *Lancet*, May 9, 1987: 1094.

[33]"Mosquitoes Do Not Spread AIDS," *The Economist*, Sept. 6, 198: 81.

[34]Lyons, S. F., et al. "Survival of HIV in the Common Bedbug," *The Lancet*, July 6, 1986: 45.

[35]Lagone 36.

[36]Lagone 49.

[37]"Sorting Out Truths from Myths"; *U.S. News and World Report* Jan. 12, 1987: 60.

[38]Amiel, B. "The Politics of a Killer Disease," *Maclean's*, Dec.8, 1986: 11.

[39]Price.

[40]Dhundale 34

[41]Fettner 64.

[42]Wahn, V., "Horizontal Transmission of HIV Infection Between Two Siblings," *The Lancet*, Sept. 20, 1986: 694.

[43]Berthier, A., "Transmissibility of Human Immunodeficiency Virus in Haemophilic and Non-haemophilic Children Living in A Private School in France," *The Lancet*, Sept. 13, 1986: 598-601.

[44]Seale, J. R. "Kuru, AIDS and Aberrant Social Behavior," *Journal of the Royal Society of Medicine*, April 1987: 202.

[45]"Science and the Citizen," *Scientific American*, Jan.1987: 58.

[46]Palca, J. "Academies Demand Urgent Public Education," *Nature* Nov. 6, 1986: 3.

[47]"What Must Be Done About AIDS?", *Nature* Nov. 6, 1986: 1.

[48]Smith, F. "AIDS Explosion is Predicted for Santa Clara County," *San Jose (California) Mercury News*, Jan. 31, 1987.

Preparation for a Plague?

The devastating effect of the AIDS virus may be due, in part, to its youth—the human body has yet to evolve a defense against it. The current state of affairs appears to indicate that this deadly disease is completely free to attack whomever it will without resistance and without compassion—it is a highly efficient, non-reasoning, killing machine. If, in the course of war, a biochemist were to develop an agent such as HIV, it would be considered the biological equivalent of nuclear weaponry in its potential destructiveness. Indeed, totally non-destructive of property, targeting only economic and social disruption, AIDS is more sophisticated than the neutron bomb.

Is a "great plague" gathering steam in the nation? Is there reason to be concerned? Unfortunately, but quite directly, the answers can only be "Yes." Robert Gallo, of the National Cancer Institute and American co-discoverer of the HIV retrovirus, calls it the "modern plague": the first great pandemic of the second half of the 20th century."[1] Dr. Halfdan Mahler stated, "We're running scared . . . we stand nakedly in front of a very serious pandemic as mortal as there has ever been. I don't know of any greater killer than AIDS, not to speak of its psychological, social and economic maiming . . . Everything is getting worse and worse in AIDS and all of us have been underestimating it."[2] Gathering force, the official projections for the next five years of the epidemic—179,000 deaths and 270,000 cumulative cases of AIDS—have been widely publicized. What is less well known, but vitally important to a logical understanding of the problem, is that those projections are certainly low. Just how low are the projections, and perhaps, even more pertinent, *why* are official projections so low? Low projections may have a critical bearing on society's perception and subsequent response—helping to insure development of the impending "modern plague."

Official Projections

The World Health Organization (WHO) estimates that as many as 5 to 10 million people around the world now carry the AIDS virus, and that as many as 100 million will become infected during the next ten years. Adding urgency to the problem of AIDS growth specifically in the United States, some epidemiologists are predicting 100,000 cases by 1988. Others estimate that as many as two million Americans may already be infected and that 400,000 people may develop AIDS over the next seven years. A potential massive number of deaths in the United States from this disease, perhaps even greater than can now be comprehended by society, is just around the corner.

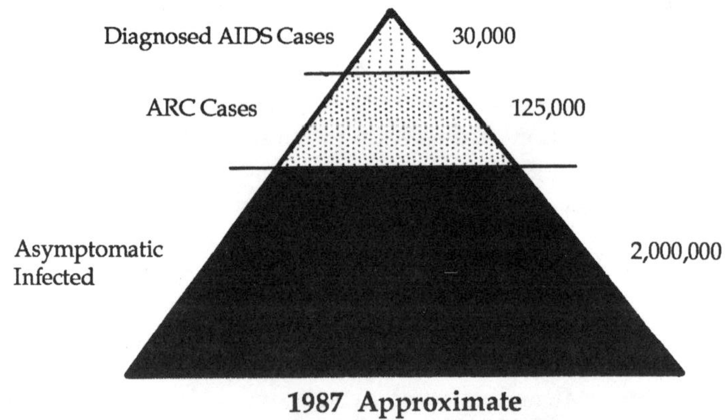

1987 Approximate
U.S. Population AIDS Data

"The AIDS Iceburg"

According to Steven L. Sivak and Gary P. Wormser of the New York Medical College there may be 300 infected American individuals for every living American adult with diagnosed AIDS, a number considerably higher than the Centers for Disease Control (CDC) figures, which estimate a 50-100 to 1 ratio. Other, more conservative, epidemiologists estimate that there may be as many as 40 to 50 unsuspecting HTLV-III/LAV carriers for every known carrier. If even the more conservative experts are right, controlling the spread of the disease will be extraordinarily difficult. Particularly disconcerting regarding estimated projections is that no one can, with any degree of scientific accuracy, state specifically how many American citizens are infected—the result of both problems of definition of the disease and valid data upon which to make predictions.

Dr. Robert Redfield, an infectious-disease specialist at the Walter Reed Army Medical Center in Washington, D.C., has stated that the AIDS virus is "likely to be present in the blood of 5 million to 10 million U.S. persons by 1991."[3] Such an estimate, given the current rate of AIDS growth, portends unparalleled national catastrophe. From 1986 to 1991, it is conceivable that there will be a 5-fold increase in the number of AIDS-infected (but not yet diagnosed) persons (1986:1.5 million—1991:7.5 million); but by 2001, a 100-fold increase of 1986 figures in the number of undiagnosed AIDS-infected persons is not beyond possibility (1986:1.5 million—1991:7.5 million—1996:37.5 million —2001:187.5 million). Clearly, a national disaster is in the making.

Efforts to Avert Disaster

United States Surgeon General C. Everett Koop, in March 1987, stated that "according to best estimates, it may not be 'until the turn of the century' before a safe and effective vaccine for AIDS is available for the general population."[4] However, Koop's estimate may be optimistic because the more we learn of the disease, the more difficult vaccine development becomes. Confounding vaccine development, "The way we see the virus now is that there aren't strains A, B, and C, but rather a continuum of virus isolates," says National Cancer Institute researcher Robert Gallo[5] and each may require its own unique vaccine.

Treatments are under development for AIDS, but those available to date have had many negative side effects and, in many cases, the treatments have been discontinued. As far as a cure for the disease is concerned, some of the best researchers in the field are very pessimistic—despite the technological sophistication of modern medicine. AIDS has, so far, shown itself to be a mystery, wrapped in an enigma. Again, HIV appears to have been designed to resist quick solution.

If science cannot solve this puzzle—or cannot solve it fast enough—the resultant number of deaths could be enormous, and all reports suggest scientists are having great difficulty unravelling the secrets of the retrovirus. Evidence currently suggests there may be sufficient justification for viewing the AIDS pandemic as the "modern plague" upon which we are, as of 1987, on the very edge. The nation has, and will continue, its movement into the AIDS era. America is totally unprepared to experience something of this magnitude in virtually all of its systems. There are no "practice runs" to decide best strageties for preparing the public or the nation's systems for what is to come and little time available for selecting choices.

AIDS Compared to the Black Death

Does AIDS possess the potential to repeat the great plagues of history and, if so, what does history have to say regarding the effects of plagues on social systems? Perhaps, of any of the historic plagues, societal experience with the Black Plague offers glimpses of what could be a possible future for the United States.

The disease occurred in the 15th year of the reign of the Roman Emperor Justinian I in A.D. 531 when, coincidentally, Halley's comet had just faded from view. Procopius, secretary of Justinian's army general Belisarius, wrote in *De bello Persico,* "the bodies of the sick were covered with black pustules or carbuncles, the symptoms of immediate death . . . Those who were without friends or servants lay unburied in the streets or in their desolate houses . . . Corpses were placed aboard ships and these abandoned to the seas . . . Physicians could not tell which cases were light and which severe, and no remedies availed."[6] By the 1300s, little had changed regarding societal response to the disease.

A most frightening plague, the "Black Death" was preceded by a series of disasters in China, beginning in 1333. There were droughts and then floods, earthquakes, and clouds of locusts blotting out the sun. Plague erupted somewhere in the East, probably in the present Kirgiz Soviet Socialist Republic and spread south and east through China and India along the major trade routes of the time. According to the *Chronica Senese,* written by Agnola di Tura during the time, "Father abandoned child; wife, husband; one brother, another; . . . And so they died. And no one could be found to bury the dead for money or for friendship . . . And I, Agnola di Tura, called the Fat, buried my five children with my own hands, and so did many others likewise."[7]

Black Death ravaged most of France in A.D. 1348 with monumental mortality—the French chronicler Jean Froissart estimated that the first wave carried off a third of the population. History records that the city of Toulouse lost nearly 50% of its population (from 40,000 to 20,000), and Normandy may have lost nearly 66% of its population during the plague years. Calculations estimating the total number dead of the population of Europe indicate 25 million persons fell victim to the Black Death.

In a famous medical treatise, French Surgeon Guy de Chauliac of Avignon recalled his impressions of the horror around him: "The father did not visit the son nor the son the father. Charity was dead and hope abandoned . . . For self-preservation there was nothing better than to flee the region before becoming infected."

Michael Platiensis of Piazza, writing an account of the plague, said, "Soon the corpses were lying forsaken in the houses. No ecclesiastic, no son, or father and no relations dared to enter, but they paid hired servants with high wages to bury the dead."[8]

Giovanni Boccaccio, writing of the Black Death in *The Decameron* said, "brother forsook brother, uncle nephew and sister brother and oftimes wife husband; nay fathers and mothers refused to visit or tend their very children, as they had not been theirs."[9] De Mussis, concerning his observations of the Black Death, wrote, "infinite number of young people, especially pregnant women died in a short time . . . the great and the noble were hurled into the same grave with the vile and the abject, because the dead were all alike."[10]

Gilles Li Muisis, abbot of St. Martin's of Tourni, France, wrote, "cattle wandering without herdsmen in the field, towns and waste-lands; that they have seen barns and wine-cellars standing wide open, houses empty and few people to be found anywhere . . . and in many different areas, both lands and fields are lying uncultivated."[11]

William of Dene, a monk of Rochester (in Kent, England) wrote, "To our great grief, the plague carried off so vast a multitude of people of both sexes that nobody could be found who would bear the corpses to the grave. Men and women carried their own children on the shoulders to the church and threw them into a common pit. From such pits such an appalling stench was given off that scarcely anyone dared even to walk beside the cemeteries. There was so marked a deficiency of labourers and workmen of every kind at this period that more than a third of the land in the whole realm was left idle. All the labourers, skilled or unskilled, were so carried away by the spirit of revolt that neither King, nor law, nor justice, could restrain them."[12] Dene continued, "in Basle the populace obliged the (police) to burn the Jews . . . Upon this, all the Jews in Basle, whose number could not have been inconsiderable, were enclosed in a wooden building, constructed for the purpose, and burnt together with it, upon the mere outcry of the people, without sentence or trial."[13]

The Great Plague of London (A.D. 1664-65) killed 15% of that city's population; the Plague of 1894, starting in China, spread across the globe killing an estimated 10 million persons worldwide. Certainly, the world is no stranger to plague, but in our late 20th-century arrogance, we have, apparently wrongly, concluded the victory over plague had been won. The present and future stark realities will remind us, once again, that we are fallible—that our ill-found arrogance may hasten a fall.

Although the AIDS "plague" is very different from the Black Death in the speed with which it kills, comparing AIDS to past killers Health and Human Services Secretary Otis Bowen stated, "If we can't make progress [against AIDS], we face the dreadful prospect of a worldwide death toll in the tens of millions a decade from now. Such earlier epidemics as typhus, small-pox and even the black death will 'look very pale by comparison.'"[14] It is absolutely imperative that the American population be informed.

In the considered opinions of some of the best scientific minds in the nation, AIDS is a national catastrophe that is already in the making. John Warden, writing in the *British Medical Journal,* said during February 1987, "So there is reason to hope that spread to the heterosexual community [in England] can be contained. The scale of the problem here is still only one tenth of what it is in the United States, even taking account of the population difference. Have we acted in time?"[15] J. Parker-Williams, consultant hematologist at St. George's Hospital Medical School in London, said, "Compared with the United States and certain countries in central Africa, the extent of the problem in the United Kingdom has so far remained small."[16] Assuming England has just acted in time and the problem is "small" (having only 10% of our AIDS problem) is it possible to deduct that we have not acted in time and our problem potentially rivals that of central Africa? Certainly, in the absence of any strategic biomolecular vaccine/treatment breakthrough, the overall numbers of potential AIDS victims far surpasses the number who died during some of the past great plagues. Clearly, the nation must mobilize its citizens to become personally involved in slowing the disease's rate of growth, yet, as of March 1987, the President of the United States and the Surgeon General were at odds regarding even a national educational strategy (Abstinence vs. 'Safe Sex') and individuals had not yet made significant changes in their sexual behavior. Denial appears to be occurring not only on an individual level, but, frighteningly, also in systems and institutions charged with the responsibility to respond.

The Physical Symptoms of AIDS

Four to 12 weeks after exposure to the virus, the infected individual may develop signs of acute infection, including prolonged fever and night sweats, extreme malaise, muscle aches, swollen lymph nodes, and rash. In most cases, these symptoms, if they do develop, resolve without complications. At that time ELISA and Western Blot tests for serum antibodies to the AIDS virus begin to show positive results indicating the presence of the virus.

Once established in the body, the virus contaminates tears and saliva. It is not proven that these fluids contain enough virus to pass the infection to another person, yet debate concerning transmission by tears and saliva continues. As the disease becomes diagnosed (which may be as long as 15 years from the initial infection), the first clinical symptoms are evident.

AIDS victims will often receive treatment for *pneumocystis carinii* pneumonia, Kaposi's sarcoma, *candidiasis, herpes zoster, cytomegalovirus, cryptococcal meningitis,* disseminate *histoplasmosis, toxoplasmosis, isosporiasis,* or any of a great number of other infections. Esophageal candidiasis may be so widespread that the patient has trouble swallowing. Additionally seen are progressive multifocal leukoencephalopathy, *cryptosporidiosis,* bronchial or pulmonary candidiasis, gastrointestinal infections, and encephalopathy.

Diseases which may be encountered by AIDS victims include: opportunistic respiratory infections experienced as rales, coughs, sneezing, and heavy bronchial secretions, and other breathing difficulties resulting in anxiety; the victim's skin may break down resulting in severe dandruff, seborrheic dermatitis, rash, ulcerated lesions of the feet, waist, or neck caused by malnutrition, fungus infections, lack of mobility, incontinence, diarrhea, herpes zoster, and Kaposi's sarcoma; debilitating diarrhea resulting in electrolyte depletion (dehydration) and lesions or other infections caused from feces; confusion, loss of memory, concentration problems, and even dementia result from AIDS's attack of the central nervous system.[17]

As of March 1986, the mean length of a person's survival after diagnosis of an AIDS-related opportunistic infection had been made was about two years and that survival time has remained relatively stable despite new treatments.

A major problem with the HTLV-III/LAV virus is that individuals infected with it can transmit the virus even if they don't develop AIDS. Persons infected by the disease may live as long as 15 (perhaps 20) years without showing any signs of its presence—the person feels and appears well. The individual continues his/her normal sexual behavior while spreading the disease. This unknowing transmission of the disease is one of its more insidious aspects and has helped its great spread in this nation. With the Black Death you knew you were infected within a day and died in three—not so with AIDS.

Can a "Plague" be Averted?

Once the magnitude of the numbers of infected individuals is truly grasped by the general population, calls for intervention will surely be made. Given a democratic society, options for effectively intervening to reduce the spread of the disease may be limited. In general terms, there are three ways to protect Americans from the virus:

1. Government could attempt to isolate or quarantine the carriers of the disease.

This strategy is already politically, ethically, and physically impossible: to develop a quarantine for those persons infected as of March 1987 would be equivalent to detaining the population of Chicago (1980 census figures: 3,005,072 million persons) and would be cost-prohibitive. Additionally, according to microbiologist David Baltimore, co-chair of the scientific panel issuing the influential status report *Confronting AIDS*, "Quarantining will help no one. Most AIDS patients are too sick to be transmitting the virus. The virus is being spread largely by people who do not have AIDS but are infected with the virus, and they may not know it. Quarantining would be futile."[18]

2. Government could attempt to identify the carriers of AIDS.

As of 1987, 21 states have enacted legislation or precedential court rulings that make AIDS a "protected handicap," further, those who reveal identifying medical information on an AIDS victim could "face tremendous potential liability to the AIDS victim, who could sue on the basis of the handicap laws, defamation, invasion of privacy, and perhaps even violation of civil rights."[19] If the government begins identification, tracking, and public labeling of AIDS victims, nothing short of suspension of civil liberties or the creation of a whole set of laws for handling the disease would be required.

3. Attempt to eliminate the common behaviors that spread the virus.

Although calls for massive public education have been made, as of March 1987 only some television networks now air public health warnings. Whether that education (media-and school-based education) will be an effective method of reducing high-risk sexual behaviors is quite another story. "A recent *NBC/Wall Street Journal* poll found that AIDS has no effect on the way 92% of the population conducts their lives even when 95% of them know what behaviors spread the disease. This is particularly true on the nation's college campuses, where sex tends to be impulsive."[20]

Other polls suggest sexual behavior is not changing. In a random survey of 800 state residents conducted by the Illinois Department of Public Health, 96% of the respondents were aware that a used hypodermic syringe could spread AIDS, 94% were aware that the virus is transmitted by having unprotected sex with an infected partner and 86% believed AIDS is likely to become an epidemic, nearly 75% admitted they had not taken any precautions to avoid the disease.

A poll conducted for *Newsweek* by the Gallop Organization in November 1986 revealed that 23% of the population felt that AIDS will not likely become an epidemic for the public at large, suggesting a relatively non-concerned public and the need for more direct education. However, even if the population is educated, no one who knows anything about sex education is willing to predict that it will make substantial changes in sexual behavior. "The number of people making real changes [in their sexual behavior to reduce risk of exposure] seems slight, even in places where information about AIDS is readily available."[21]

An editorial in the *American Journal of Public Health* gives warning: "Nevertheless, one cannot help but be skeptical about the magnitude of any long-term impact of such [educational] efforts in the light of past experience with sexually transmitted diseases."[22] Education without effort to impress the absolute reality of the impact of this disease upon both individuals and society may be ineffective.

In regard to education of school children, a survey released during January 1987 by the U. S. Conference of Mayors of the nation's 74 largest school districts found that 40 districts provide AIDS education programs of some sort and 23 others will do so by Fall 1987.[23] Despite this belated incorporation of AIDS education into the classroom, "experts say the message about AIDS is not getting through; in some cases because of a lack of available information and in others because young people simply aren't listening."[24] Dr. June Osborn, of the University of Michigan, said, "the youth audience must be informed if disaster is to be prevented. It's particularly important that we reach adolescents because they are still in the process of establishing behavior patterns."[25] Dr. Evelyn Fischer of the infectious diseases department at Ford Hospital, Detroit, Michigan, said quite bluntly, "This country has two choices: either we grow up and talk about it, or we watch our children and grandchildren get AIDS."[26]

As AIDS touches more and more aspects of everyday life—the education of children, marriage rites, sexual habits, health care and insurance—AIDS will transform American society. "By 1991," says Michael Gottlieb, the physician at the University of California, Los Angeles who identified some of the first cases of the disease, "most people in certain cities will know someone who has died of AIDS."[27] Dr. Robert Gallo stated in the January 1987 *Scientific American*, "Yet even if therapy and vaccine are brought into being on the fastest possible schedule, HTLV-III's toll will be heavy: many of the millions already infected will become ill before treatment is available." It is certain that AIDS will change the nation—just how and when changes occur will become increasingly important as numbers escalate.

As mentioned earlier, relying on the scientific establishment to develop the "magic bullet" appears foolish. Apart from the unique problems posed by the virus itself, the pragmatic barriers to testing, licensing and marketing a vaccine are staggering: large groups of healthy subjects willing to be innoculated with a potentially lethal virus, issues of liability to be faced, decisions as to whether to target groups and so stigmatize them, or to recommend universal use and face a situation comparable to that of swine flu may prohibit rapid vaccine development. In the absence of an effective cure or vaccine, what, then, do the next 15-25 years hold—given the already widely spread viral invasion and with both the population and responsible institutions denying the magnitude of the threat.

A prudent strategy appears to be not only education to stem the disease's spread but, additionally, societal sexual behavior changes in the advent of delayed/no effective vaccine or treatment. To hope that education will change individuals' or institutions' behavior without their having an appreciation for the possible consequences if they do not change—not only to themselves, but to the nation—is whistling in the dark.

Storm Clouds on the Horizon

Certainly those in authority are capable of reducing the potential for spreading the disease and leading the nation through the crisis—or are they? In the coming years, as the AIDS epidemic gathers momentum, there is going to be an interesting interplay of logic and emotion. "It will be a curious period for us all. . . . Somehow it will be necessary to combine a sense of urgency with a sense of the importance of civility that makes society worthwhile. The danger is that some will be overwhelmed by the urgency."[28] Hints of panic are beginning to be seen: the public wants guidelines and new rules for unprecedented circumstances. The extremely optimistic medical consensus is that a means of arresting AIDS will come no sooner than five or ten years, suggesting potential problems. Other authorities, including Robert C. Gallo, suggest that a means of arresting the disease *may never come.*

As is becoming increasingly evident, "scientific facts" are wrought with inconsistencies, contradictions, and frequent changes as more is learned. For example, in 1985, "some scientists made flimsy cases for the imminent spread of the disease (AIDS) into the heterosexual population. They cited vague and unverifiable statistics about men who contracted AIDS from female prostitutes, and made reference to the high incidence of the disease among purported heterosexuals in central Africa,"[29] but in 1987 the consensus is, "We're not saying there is an epidemic in the heterosexual population right now. But when you have an infectious pool as large as a million people, I think the risk is enormous. If we ignore this potential, we're doing it at great risk to everybody."[30] Are the "facts" that are currently being reported to the public true or are the "facts" subject to two-year revisions?

Suggesting that heterosexual transmission of the disease is a reality, recently (March 1987) compiled U. S. military statistics find that the ratio of infected men to infected women in their study is about 2.5 to 1, a great contrast to the estimated national average of about 13 infected men for every 1 infected woman. Donald Burke of the Walter Reed Army Medical Center reports that the AIDS virus is transmitted very efficiently through normal heterosexual contact. In fact, reports from the May 31 - June 5, 1987 Washington D. C. International AIDS Conference suggest AIDS is spreading at twice the speed through the heterosexual population than it did through the homosexual population.

To further raise concern about "facts" and reality, "There is a growing list of cell types the AIDS virus can infect"—those of the monocyte/macrophage type—including "Langerhans cells in the skin (cells in the outer (epidermis) skin), lung macrophages (can the virus, if airborne through aerosol, enter the body through this route?), brain macrophages (as many as 66% of AIDS patients develop dementia), and follicular dendritic cells (nerve cells at the base of hairs) in the lymph nodes. It is also possible that the virus infects some B-lymphocytes, brain astrocytes and microglia (both structurally integral to brain shape, size, and function), and T8 cells that have been transformed by a different human retrovirus, HTLV-I."[31] Evidence presented later suggests HTLV-I may be as problematic as AIDS in the near future. Do any of these recent findings have any effect on the reality of the "fact" that infection through casual contact is not possible? What will be the consensus in two years?

The degree to which scientific facts are changing or raising the level of public concern without touching off hysteria is the key to both the credibility of the public health-complex and an understanding of the magnitude of the problem. Britain's Secretary of State for Health and Social Services, Norman Fowler said in a January 1987 meeting with San Francisco health officials, "The most important thing we have to do is convince people of the urgency of the situation without causing personal alarm and panic."[32] However, without a realistic understanding of the potential of the AIDS epidemic, individual sexual behavior is not likely to change. Maybe even more damaging is the fact that the American public may loose faith in the honesty of the public health network, an event certain to diminish its long term influence.

Changing a Nation's Sexual Behavior

"In general, the higher the degree of risk that can be projected for a particular individual, the easier it is to affect his behavior. The perception of a high risk and a catastrophic outcome might be expected to induce the greatest motivation to change, while a low risk and a negligible outcome should have little impact. When the perceived risk involved is as low as it is for most heteroxsexuals thinking about AIDS [as they and public educational strategies continue to deny the reality of this disease], the perceived severity of the outcome may not matter."[33] From a strictly behavioral standpoint, current informational approaches appear flawed—insuring both a credibility gap for both the public health and mass media systems as well as an increased percentage of the general population being infected.

If substantial reality-based public education is not provided and should AIDS spread in the most pessimistic proportions projected with millions being infected, there may finally sound a general alert, resulting in an increase in monogamy, in abstinence, and in widespread acceptance of the destructive power of AIDS (and subsequent political backlash). But unless and until that point comes, casualties may needlessly mount. Recent information from testing of military recruits shows that the disease is likely to be transmitted at an increasing rate within the general population in the United States, setting a potential for eventual panic.

Dr. Eskild A. Petersen, an infectious-disease expert at the University of Arizona, said in January 1987, "The numbers of cases are clearly going way up. I didn't used to be so pessimistic. But it is clear now that AIDS is going to overshadow any other disease we've ever had to handle. The numbers [of AIDS cases] in this state and nation-wide are now beginning to follow the worst predictions we had heard. I didn't used to buy those predictions. But the numbers now are so great, and our behavior is basically unchanged. It will be impossible to keep AIDS down."[34]

The very "hysteria" which authorities are now trying to avert may, in the long run, lead to an even more explosive social upheaval. Frankly stated, why aren't those charged with protecting society doing so? Dr. Neil Schram, chairman of the Los Angeles AIDS task force, stated that if an effective vaccine is not developed, "society will be divided—not between gays and nongays, but between those who are infected and those who are not infected."

He continued, "the likelihood of a successful medical solution, like a vaccine or a cure, and the political demands . . . will inevitably lead to the disruption of our free society."[35] Just what these "disruptions" may be, how they may develop, and what can be done to mitigate their impact is increasingly important as the scientific community continues to push "effective vaccine/cure" development into the future. We are headed into uncharted waters and no hand appears to be on the rudder.

Epilogue

That AIDS holds the potential for repeating the "Black Death" is virtually assured in central Africa, even if a vaccine is developed tomorrow. Whether a repeat or an approximation of the plague can result from AIDS in the United States hinges on a number of variables, many of which are not well understood.

Despite reports of vaccine development it may not be until the turn of the century before an effective vaccine is available. Until (or if) a vaccine/cure is developed, projections of AIDS in the United States continue to become more grim. By 1991 a con-servative estimate shows cumulative AIDS deaths in the U.S. at 175,000 persons (a tenfold increase in 5 years); by 2001, deaths in that single year may be 1.5 million with 50 million Americans infected by the virus.

Educational methods are not likely to affect individual sexual behavior until the disease epidemic becomes much worse. It is not unlikely that profound social, institutional, and political changes may occur. Denial of the potential impact of the disease seems to be occurring not only by individuals but by institutions responsible for averting such an impact at a time when stark reality must be faced.

In the following pages, the potential impact of AIDS on the medical, insurance, social welfare, federal government, and legal/constitutional systems will be explored. Additionally, the impact of AIDS on the social fabric of the nation, AIDS vaccines and treatment, and a general summary will be presented. The intent in the exploration of AIDS's impact is to establish potentials which may occur and that, therefore, can be anticipated, controlled or prevented.

Notes

[1]Gallo, R. C. "The AIDS Virus," *Scientific American*, 256.1: 47.

[2]Antonio, G. THE AIDS COVER-UP? (San Francisco: Ignatius Press, 1987) 239.

[3]Morganthau, T., et al. "The AIDS Epidemic: Future Shock," *Newsweek*, November 24, 1986: 31.

[4]*Face the Nation*, National Broadcasting Company, March 29, 1987.

[5]Dusheck, J. "HTLV-III Virus: Themes and Variations," *Science News*, 128.8: 119.

[6]Gregg, Charles T. PLAGUE (New York: Charles Scribner's Sons, 1978) 5.

[7]Gregg 7.

[8]Marks, G. M., et al. EPIDEMICS (New York: Charles Scribner's Sons, 1976) 76.

[9]Marks 80.

[10]Marks 83.

[11]Marks 85.

[12]Marks 86.

[13]Marks 90.

[14]*Summit Journal*, March 1987.

[15]Warden, J. "The Politics of AIDS," *British Medical Journal*, Feb. 14, 1987: 455.

[16]Parker-Williams, J. "Our Response to AIDS," *Journal of the Royal Society of Medicine*, May 1987: 264.

[17]Coleman, D. A. "How to Care for an AIDS Patient," *RN*, July 1986: 16-18.

[18]"Quarantining Will Help No One," an interview with AIDS expert and Nobel laureate David Baltimore, *U.S. News and World Report* Jan. 12, 1987: 70.

[19]Rowe, M. P., et al. "The Fear of AIDS," *Harvard Business Review*, July-Aug. 1986: 34.

[20]Smilgis, Martha. "The Big Chill: Fear of AIDS," *Time*, Feb. 16, 1987: 52

[21]Leishman, K. "Heterosexuals and AIDS," *Atlantic Monthly*, Feb. 1987: 44.

[22]Yankauer, A. "The Persistence of Public Health Problems," *AJPH*, 76 . 5: 495.

[23]Marklewicz, D. "Young People Ignore Threat, Survey Finds," *Detroit (Michigan) News*, Feb. 3, 1987.

[24]Marklewicz.

[25]Marklewicz.

[26]Marklewicz.

[27]Wallis, C. "You Haven't Heard Anything Yet," *Time*, Feb. 16, 1987: 56.

[28]"What Must Be Done About AIDS?," *Nature*, Nov. 6, 1986. 1.

[29]Langone, J. AIDS: Special Report, *Discover* 6.12(1985): 30.

[30]Zimmerman, D. R., et al. "Complete Medical Report," *McCall's*, 114. 7(1987): 14.

[31]Barnes, D. M. "The Complexity of the AIDS Virus,"*Science*. 233.4761: 282.

[32]Palmer, M. "British Health Chief Visits S.F. in War on AIDS," *San Francisco (California) Examiner*, Jan. 19, 1987.

[33]Leishman, K. "Heterosexuals and AIDS," *The Atlantic Monthly*, Feb. 1987: 41.

[34]McClain, C. "Deadly Disease's Numbers 'Galloping,' Expert Says Here," *Tucson (Arizona) Citizen*, Jan. 29, 1987.

[35]Morganthau 31.

The Impact of AIDS on the Medical System

As the epidemic continues its exponential advance, it poses an economic threat to the United States. The cost of caring for victims of the disease, many of whom are denied health insurance, is already estimated to exceed a billion dollars a year. Dr. Ann Hardy of the CDC said in 1987, "The first 424 cases of AIDS in children in the United States have cost $25 million in direct health care costs, including hospitalization and nursing care."[1] By 1991 estimates of AIDS medical bills range from as little as $8.5 billion to as much as $14 billion annually. In Santa Clara County, California alone, the costs of providing medical care to patients in 1991 could reach $144 million (annually) and the cumulative costs could be much greater. Estimates for California in 1991 range between $255-$406 million.

Donald McDonald, assistant secretary of health of the Public Health Service, stated "In 1991 the medical care of AIDS patients [nationally] will require between $8 and $16 billion [based on the assumptions that the average cost per patient will be about $46,000 and the CDC projections are accurate]," an amount not including home care given by friends or family or lost income due to illness.[2] Many studies show that the average medical cost per AIDS patient is approximately $147,000.

Signs of Stress

"I don't see how the existing system can continue to care for AIDS patients without compromising other groups of patients," said Paul Volberding, director of the AIDS program at San Francisco General Hospital. To help alleviate the situation, he proposed that national regional hospitals, specializing in the care of AIDS patients, be developed. Further, both he and David Werdegar, Director of the San Francisco Department of Health, strongly advocate direct federal government involvement in planning short- and long-term responses to the AIDS epidemic.

Werdegar stated: "The government ought to have a national commission that is looking in a coordinated way at what is a national emergency."

The concern expressed by Volberding and Werdegar is not unfounded. In the absence of a cure/vaccine for AIDS, "by 1991 the number of total AIDS patients in San Francisco may be close to 18,000, a number 2 to 3 times the 8000 cases predicted by the Centers for Disease Control.[3] *BusinessWeek* quotes Volberding, saying "I have some real concerns as to where we are going to care for these people" and, at the annual meeting of the American Association for the Advancement of Science in February 1987, he stressed, "The San Francisco model works for now but (will) not in the future." A Santa Clara County California taskforce report stated in 1987 that theye are now feeling the initial wave of what will be the worst epidemic ever experienced by the medical professions in the county.

Perhaps as a forewarning of AIDS treatment and medical service delivery problems, the San Francisco system has experienced a high incidence of absenteeism, turnover, and burnout among treatment staff, and the replacement of volunteers is becoming more difficult.[4] Ron Rose of Being Alive, a coalition of AIDS patients, speaking in February 1987 of the AIDS ward at Los Angeles County-USC Medical Center, said the facility is "overcrowded, understaffed and the rate of burn-out is incredibly high—anyone with AIDS would rather die at home than die at USC."[5] Since, in 1991, the AIDS epidemic by even the most conservative estimates may be one of the worst epidemics in U.S. history, it is apparent that the American medical system, both people and facilities, will be challenged as never before. It has been reported that in New York City and Newark, New Jersey "pediatric AIDS cases already have sorely taxed those areas' health care systems, and there still are not very many efforts under way there or elsewhere in the nation to cope with the thousands of childhood AIDS cases that will be seen by the end of the decade."[6] Crisis management is the order of the day in many medical facilities.

Can Effective Adjustments Be Made?

"At present, state and local health services are largely unequipped to cope with sharply rising numbers of persons infected with the AIDS virus or sick with the full disease [requiring] greatly expanded educational and training programs for health-care workers."[7] Also, if either out-patient or home-based treatment is to be used as a means to reduce patient care costs, which is likely, the visiting-nurse programs in many cities are hardly prepared for the immense needs or number of patients who are or will be dying of AIDS. Many patients may require 24-hour care by skilled professionals.

In an effort to begin provision for training, The National Institute of Mental Health began in August 1986 reviewing contract proposals to develop training programs for health-care personnel on mental health issues related to AIDS. The programs are designed to educate nurses, doctors, and other health-care professionals now in training, and will be available to those health professionals already in practice and to nonprofessional health-care workers who counsel AIDS patients.

Three new bills have been introduced in Congress, with at least a fourth in preparation, to establish a national coordinating body to combat AIDS. Still being drafted is a separate bill from Senator Edward Kennedy (D-MA) that will include additional money for AIDS research outside the existing NIH budget, as well as more funds for education and public health. The Kennedy bill will also try to create an environment that will foster the development of a vaccine to prevent AIDS. The appropriate questions appear to be: will training programs be funded at a sufficient level?; will these programs provide training to a sufficient number of persons to deliver effective services to infected individuals?; will these training programs reach sufficient numbers of lower-level health service technicians to meet AIDS's exponential growth?; will that training be, in reality, capable of producing any but the most superficial impact?; and, can the Federal Government continue to provide ever-increasing funding?

Breakdown in Health Care?

As an example of problems to come, Peter Ungvarski, Cabrini Medical Center, reported incidents of improper care delivered to AIDS patients. "I saw one case where *Candidia* had been allowed to build up in a patient's mouth to the point where we were pulling it out like cottage cheese." Ungvarski continued, "Another time I visited a patient at home after he'd been treated for meningitis in another hospital [but] his coordination was so bad he couldn't empty his own indwelling chemo catheter [and no one] had bothered to assess him after his meningitis [for] residual neurological defects."

Other reports of hospitalized AIDS patients left languishing, of food trays hastily placed outside patients' doors, and cans of nutritional supplement stacking up in patients' rooms are not unknown. In some hospitals, "AIDS patients are being placed in the same rooms or wards with immuno-compromised non-AIDS patients (cancer and/or transplant patients) without the latter being informed. This is an unethical and dangerous violation of the protocol called for in treating AIDS patients."[8]

What Can Be Done?

If AIDS develops to the potential A.D. 2001 projections and if health-care costs per patient remain near $49,000, a total annual AIDS health-care expenditure of $73.5-$147 billion per year may not be unrealistic—an amount approximately equal to the total U.S. Federal Budget as recently as the late '60s. Health-care costs could well be $250-600 billion per year if costs per patient are closer to $147,000—approximately half of the total 1987 Federal Budget. From where will those funds come?

As a result of these projected drastic increases in costs, some health planners foresee much wider use of alternative-care facilities for AIDS patients—hospices, nursing homes and in-home care by visiting nurses. It will apparently be necessary for hospitals to serve AIDS patients in acute medical crisis only, and the epidemic's other victims will receive less intensive care elsewhere. This approach, described by Dr. John Mills, chief of infectious diseases at San Francisco General Hospital, as "Machiavellian," is based on the financial exigencies posed by AIDS's predicted explosive growth. Yet, whether patient payment for these "less intensive" services will remain feasible is open to debate.

It appears that, in the face of a projected onslaught of cases, new care facilities will be necessary. Where funding will come from for additional hospices, nursing homes, and/or national regional hospitals specializing in the care of AIDS patients, is questionable. If the Federal government is expected to contribute funding for development of these facilities at the same time the tax base (through illness and death) is decreasing, either a reprioritization of federal funds, an increase in the national debt, an increase in taxes, or a disruption of health-care services will be required. If additional facilities are to be constructed without or with minimal Federal support, then increases in either AIDS patients' or all patients' health-care costs seems probable.

An increased need for funds (regardless of source) for development of new facilities is occurring, and shall contine to occur, at a time when a need for increased funding for health care staff and skilled expertise is evident. Further, as cases skyrocket, the rate at which these new staff shall be required suggests either a re-assignment of present staff (which would surely decrease levels of care to other patient groups) or a hasty addition of new staff, which may result in insufficient training, resulting in substandard care for AIDS patients. In any planned transition from re-assigned staff to the addition of new staff, a decreased level of care for both patient groups may occur. Certainly the process of staff training in the provision of health-care services to AIDS patients will, of necessity, be a continuing and escalating process—translating into additional costs. Perhaps both Federal and State welfare recipients will be "drafted" as health-care providers as a method of containing escalating costs.

A Possible Scenario?

In the provision of medical/health care services in the face of the expected AIDS catastrophe, this A.D. 2001 scenario appears a possibility:

> Virtually every hospital in the nation has, as a significant percentage of its outpatients, ARC or AIDS-infected individuals who are in the early stages of the disease. The nationalized hospice and regional AIDS-care hospital systems, an outgrowth of nationalized health insurance since 1994, have been providing non-heroic care—the centers have become a 'place to die' and are greatly feared by the general population.
>
> Reminiscent of early 20th century mental health care, staffing of hospice and regional-care centers is a continual problem; staff turnover, improper training and treatment, patient abuse (both physical and mental), and staff-assisted patient suicide are

> rumored. Daily patient intake and removal of the dead have taken a heavy emotional toll on staff and the rate of suicide among health-care professionals has increased. The number of persons entering into the health-care professions, which shows remarkable growth in the early 1990's, has begun to decline significantly as a result of deteriorating morale.
>
> The specter of additional millions soon to enter the medical system continues to dwarf current health-care capabilities and a pattern of crisis-management is routinr. It is clearly apparent to planners that, without major federal support (both technical and monetary), the system will fail. Yet that support will likely not come. A call for military support has been considered.

Again, science fiction? Perhaps not. Dr. Renslow Sherer Jr., director of the Cook County Hospital AIDS program in Chicago, says, "The implications [of the 1991 projections of AIDS] are staggering. At Cook County we would need . . . almost a whole wing devoted to these people. We'll need psycho-social support, emotional care, resources for abandoned and homeless patients. And we're probably talking about a *diversion* of resources from other areas."[9] A 1987 Santa Clara California taskforce report (1987) outlined 37 recommendations for meeting the medical, social service, educational, psychological and housing needs of AIDS patients. This report of only *one county,* hints at health care problems to come. Ken Yeager, chairman of the Santa Clara County Taskforce, said, "The AIDS projections are staggering. . . ." The House of Commons (England) Social Services Committee has generated a report on AIDS and emerged with a list of 94 recommendations and conclusions regarding planning for sufficient resources of money, manpower, facilities, and training to ensure that the health and social services can cope with the demands put upon them.[10]

"At this point, real planning for the crisis that lies ahead has barely begun: if AIDS is war, the policymakers who command the health-care army are pushing paper regiments across blurry maps of a world they can only dimly foresee."[11] Unless, or until, the medical community mobilizes to fight an epidemic of the magnitude of the European "black death," crisis management, replete with its pitfalls, seems assured. Even if mobilization occurs, expected funding difficulties portend solutions radically different from tradition. Unfortunately, but realistically, it may be too late to avert a breakdown in the American health-care system.

Epilogue

That the medical establishment will face an unprecedented challenge in the delivery of health-care services to the nation's AIDS-infected population is certain. Virtually assured to become reality, 1991 projections in several larger cities when they materialize will create problems of both patient housing and trained staffing of facilities. If a cure/vaccine is not available by 2001, the medical community will be faced with what could be a nightmare scenario of burgeoning patient-load, inadequate facilities, untrained and/or severely emotionally distressed staff, and no hope for substantial funding. It is not beyond reason to expect that the nation's health-care system may come unraveled.

If national health care insurance is not effected, health-care costs will certainly skyrocket. Further, at a time when additional health-care staff are most needed, the number of persons entering the field will be greatly reduced—a result of morale problems from massive deaths. Continued hope of a cure/vaccine must remain. The health-care community must greatly increase staff training, facilities, and public education, lobby for nationalized health insurance, and create alternatively-funded, community-based health-care cooperatives. If this is not done, we may see a health-care panic. Because of the massive federal debt, substantial federal support may not materialize.

Notes

[1]Biner, D. "House OKs Bill Aimed at Halting AIDS Spread," *(Atlanta, Georgia) Journal* Feb. 21, 1987.

[2]Barnes, D. M. "AIDS Stresses Health Care in San Francisco," *Science* 235.4792: 964.

[3]Barnes 964.

[4]"Volunteers, Home Care, and Money: How San Francisco Has Mobilized," *Business Week*, March 23, 1987: 125.

[5]Hastings, D. "AIDS Care Called a 'Scandal' During Plea for L.A. Hospices," *Los Angeles (California) Herald Examiner*, Feb. 17, 1987.

[6]Biner.

[7]Barnes, D. M. "Grim Projections for AIDS Epidemic," *Science* 232. 4758: 1590.

[8]Antonio, G. THE AIDS COVER-UP? (San Francisco: Ignatius Press, 1987) 136.

[9]Morganthau, T., et al. "The AIDS Epidemic: Future Shock," *Newsweek* Nov. 24, 1986: 33-34.

[10]"Third Report from the Social Services Committee," House of Commons, Session 1986-1987, Problems associated with AIDS, May 13, 1987.

[11]Morganthau 33.

The Impact of AIDS on the Insurance System

The insurance industry, of economic necessity, must adjust quickly to the potential realities of the AIDS epidemic in America. According to Dr. Donald C. Chambers, vice president and chief medical director for Lincoln National Life, "The insurance industry in general and the underwriting profession in particular have been placed in a precarious position as a result of the AIDS epidemic."[1] A 1987 statement issued by the American Academy of Actuaries criticizing state laws which ban screening practices for AIDS cautioned, "Regulators should carefully consider the consequences of prohibiting the use of these [ELISA and Western Blot HTLV-III blood serum] tests. Such legislation could seriously affect the financial soundness of the private insurance system, the overall fairness of the risk classification system, and the availability of insurance coverage to the public."[2]

An Actuarial Nightmare

The American Council of Life Insurance reports that "those who test positive for AIDS antibodies have a 20 times greater chance of dying within five years than those who do not," and many of the nation's insurance companies "such as Aetna, John Hancock, and Metropolitan, require the AIDS antibody test as a prerequisite for some types of individual health and life insurance policies."[3] According to the American Academy of Actuaries, individuals with AIDS antibodies cannot be considered insurable because of their high mortality rate which "appears to greatly exceed the 500% of standard level which has proved to be the practical limit of substandard mortality that can be insured."[4]

Insurance companies now (March 1987) requiring blood tests to determine the presence of antibodies to the AIDS virus are drawing criticism of discrimination from gay activists.

Some cities and states have banned blood antibody testing. Arguing for the National Gay Rights Association of San Francisco, Attorney Benjamin Schatz remarked (March 1987), "If they're [insurance companies] allowed to test for this illness, it could result in massive testing for all kinds of ailments —millions of people could be denied vital health insurance, and the taxpayers would be picking up massive bills. It could set a dangerous precedent."[5] Attorney Jim Kellogg, of the Lambda Legal Defense and Education Fund, Inc. of New York, remarked in February, 1987, "The scariest part of all is that test information goes to a centralized computer bank which any insurance company can check—the person may never be able to buy insurance. It's a horrible problem."[6]

Insurance Companies Respond

Some companies, in an effort to reduce their financial risks, have ceased providing life insurance in those areas where tests are banned, e. g., in Washington, D. C., where an estimated 80% of the 600 insurance companies in business there no longer write policies. Currently California and Wisconsin do not allow insurance firms to screen applicants for AIDS antibodies. Dr. Robert Gleeson, Northwestern Mutual Life's medical director, and Russel Iuculano, American Council of Life Insurance legislative director, have argued that if AIDS victims are exempt from the usual rules of insurability, then rates will go up for other policy holders and some marginal insurance companies could even become insolvent.

Other companies, in an attempt to circumvent blood testing difficulties, ask potential insurees if they have been diagnosed as having AIDS, AIDS Related Complex (ARC) or an immune disorder. Spokesperson for Lincoln National Life Insurance Company Gerald Davis says, "It's [asking the AIDS question] part of our standard application. If someone says yes, it doesn't preclude life insurance, but we then ask for more medical information." In fact asking potential insurees their AIDS-status is done by nearly half of the companies writing life insurance in the United States.[7]

David E. Gooding, executive vice-president for individual insurance at Transamerica Occidental Life Insurance, has stated "the category of people who have a poor T-cell count are rejected as a class."[8] Geoff Wilkinson, spokesman for the New Orleans Life Insurance Underwriters Association, stated that the insurance industry is a discriminatory industry, but we discriminate across the board. It's easy for the public to see us as the big, bad insurance company. We're certainly not trying to be discriminatory, but we've been doing business for years based on our ability to classify risks."[9]

Discriminatory Insurance and Ethics Problems?

In California, National Gay Rights Advocates has filed a $10-million sex-discrimination suit against Great Republic Life Insurance, charging that the company has decided to refuse coverage to unmarried males working in such occupations as antique dealer, florist and consultant. Perhaps factors used in the choice of potential insurees are, de facto, discriminatory, yet the manner in which a judgement to insure is made must be based on more valid evidence than a person's occupation. Such strategies are, quite simply, ridiculous.

Of further concern to persons diagnosed with AIDS, some insurance companies are 'dumping' patients because of the enormous costs involved. Director of Houston's Institute for Immunological Disorders Dr. Peter Mansell has remarked that 30 percent of insurance claims filed by AIDS patients at his hospital are rejected because insurers claim they are pre-existing disorders. Appeals litigation directed toward overcoming perceived discrimination against AIDS patients in this situation is often slow to progress through the courts. Companies, according to Benjamin Schatz, director of the National Gay Rights Advocates' AIDS Civil Rights Project, bank on the fact that the life-span of the typical lawsuit is longer than the life-span of the typical person with AIDS.

Insurance Companies and Confidentiality

Another concern raised against blood testing and the insurance industry is the issue of confidentiality. "Unlike other kinds of information to which underwriters have access, antibody test information, if leaked, could conceivably lead to loss of job, loss of housing and even loss of family and friends"[10] Even though the insurance industry does take great care in maintaining confidentiality some companies may share information with medical information bureaus. These bureaus serve as a clearinghouse for medical information on clients from which insurance companies may access client medical information.

Additionally, even if extreme care is taken that information be strictly confidential any guarantee does not preclude theft of that information. Certainly insurance companies must, in underwriter efforts to reduce risk, design systems which absolutely prevent theft and/or misappropriation of client information before blood testing gains states' legislative support. Further, the practice of sharing medical information with medical information bureaus is a factor mitigating against acceptance of blood testing and an area which must be seriously addressed by the insurance industry if it intends to gain support from the general population.

Economic Impacts

Whether the projected AIDS epidemic will greatly affect the financial solvency of the life insurance industry is debatable. The American Council of Life Insurance reported that the first 1,024 death claims from AIDS have cost insurers about $34.2 million. Insurance companies are prudently attempting to minimize financial expenditure, as they should, but at what potential social costs? Assuming a $25,000 life insurance policy on only half of the potential AIDS victims in A.D. 2001, collective costs to insurers may approach $18.75 billion, an amount equal to only .34% of the life insurance in force in the U. S. in 1984.[11] In a worse scenario, where 10 million Americans insured each at $100,000 die, collective costs to insurers may approach $1 trillion, or only 18.2% of the life insurance in force as of 1984. If any of these scenarios occur in the out-years (i.e., 2010), the life insurance industry could face seriously eroded capital *if* the industry continues AIDS death benefits.

Christopher Noblet, a speech writer for Transamerica Occidental Life Insurance Company of Los Angeles, stated in 1987 that "life insurance claims to date are not an astronomical amount, but we're most worried about our future claims when the number of deaths will be much higher."[12] William F. Buckley, in a 1987 editorial estimated that potential medical costs for AIDS patients could be $10 trillion if AIDS deaths go unchecked and devastate the U. S. population.[10]

Dr. Donald Chambers of Lincoln National Life remarked, "The final question is who is going to pay for the high costs of this epidemic? In this age of budgetary cutbacks, many state lawmakers believe that insurance companies, rather than taxpayers, should foot this bill—at least for the time being." Chambers continued, "This reasoning fails to recognize that insurers already are paying a substantial share of the cost under the terms of existing contracts. Adding to the cost shifting that already is occurring will unfairly harm the vast majority of policyowners and stockholders, all of whom are taxpayers."[14]

The only financially prudent decision for insurers is to cease life and health insurance of any/all groups/individuals potentially at high risk for AIDS now so as to avoid precedential problems later—but at what eventual social cost? Those companies which are not now reducing their risks will certainly need to closely watch those companies which are reducing risks, since, as the numbers of infected grow, there will be a gravitation away from testing insurers to non-testing insurers. This shifting selection of potential insurers will most surely disproportionately increase their risks. Denial of insurance is certainly an appropriately prudent financially-based decision but one with potentially major social impact as more heads-of-households die leaving an economically disrupted family.

Government and the Insurance Crisis

Government may have to step in where underwriters fear to tread. Of 325 insurance companies surveyed in 1985, 91% refused to issue health insurance policies to people who test positive on the AIDS blood tests. Without health insurance, few Americans can handle the estimated $60,000 to $75,000 (now closer to $147,000) lifetime costs of treatment for AIDS, and most AIDS patients are not immediately eligible for Medicare or Medicaid. Yet, according to the *Washington (D. C.) Times*, "Proposed cuts in Federal 1987 Medicaid payments could seriously hurt AIDS patients unless state and local governments finance the difference."[15] If William F. Buckley's remark of a possible $10 trillion expense is anywhere near accurate it is doubtful that even the federal government will be capable of assistance.

Attempts to spread the potential economic risk across states for AIDS treatment have begun. "Eleven states have created risk pools that guarantee coverage to people whose applications for insurance [have been] refused. The pools take in people with all sorts of problems, not just those who appear to be at risk for AIDS. Premiums under such pooling arrangements [however] run to about 150% of the average rates for individuals."[16] As the projected number of AIDS patients geometrically rises, those state health insurance pools may, of necessity, need to raise premiums to a point where they become unaffordable, are subsidized by redistribution or increases of state funds, or cease to exist—state health insurance pools appear a short-term solution.

Employee Health Insurance and AIDS

"Much of the burden [of increased health care costs] will fall on corporations: 70% of the population has health insurance provided by employers, who typically pay about 80% of the cost; the [(increased) costs (will)] hit the insurer first, but then the employer's premium goes up."[17] To what extent increased health insurance premiums will affect employer provision of health benefits to employees is not known. In smaller companies it is not unlikely that provision of employee health insurance will cease. The American Academy of Actuaries has indicated that the effects of AIDS on group life insurance may be relatively small. However, effects on group health insurance may result in stricter underwriting practices or increased coverage limitations. Smaller groups' and larger groups' premiums will hinge on the numbers of claims by the group.[18] Smaller companies having a health insurance benefit may find difficulties ahead—"Just a few AIDS cases can negate the savings painfully achieved through several years of strenuous effort at benefit cost containment. In a smaller company the burden may be cataclysmic."[19]

Frightening Prospects

Inevitably, as the epidemic advances, it appears that any

current or anticipated method of assisting patients will eventually fail. This potential failure may result in large numbers of persons without any type of medical service. Conceivably, at some point, starting with the poor and eventually creeping up the economic ladder, government-supported euthanasia may be the result.

Epilogue

An AIDS epidemic will effect the insurance industry as has nothing else in its history. If projected AIDS numbers materialize it would not be unlikely that, by popular demand, a nationalized health insurance program will be discussed. Whether one is created depends upon other national economic factors: the national debt and deficit. In the absence of some type of health insurance system to provide the costs of care for AIDS victims, hospitalization and other health-care costs can be expected to rise astronomically. Many victims will be unable to afford treatment, forcing those of the non-infected population, in effect, to subsidize victims' care through increased insurance costs. It may be likely that smaller corporations, pressed by increasing employee health insurance benefits, may cease providing health insurance. Political instability resulting from exorbitant insurance and health care costs may develop.

If death benefits for AIDS victims are either denied or not available because of non-insurability, economic instability appears likely for survivors, resulting in real estate foreclosures and defaulted loans. The number of "new poor," homeless, and destitute may rise, further straining social "safety net" services. Whether insurance companies and employee health benefits programs will be financially stressed by the AIDS epidemic is unknown. The effect will be based on whether prudent business practices occur. However, social disruption, caused by a lack of both health and life insurance protection and subsequent economic displacement may need to be resolved by the nationalization of the health/life insurance industry. Cautious decision-making by the insurance industry, employers, investors, and government is absolutely necessary.

The potential extrapolation of trends suggests that any currently available method of medical/life insurance, whether corporate or state, may fail, resulting in an ethical re-evaluation of euthanasia. That the poor and minorities will first be affected by any ethical shift seems assured.

Notes

[1]Chambers, D. C. "A Prudent Approach to AIDS Testing," *Best's Review*, Sept.1986: 19.

[2]"Actuaries Join the Call to Permit AIDS Screening," *Best's Review* 6.

[3]Hamilton, J. O., et al. "The AIDS Epidemic and Business," *Businessweek*, March 23, 1987: 124.

[4]"Actuaries" 6.

[5]Booker, L. D. "Insurance Firms Test, Reject Applicants Exposed to AIDS," *(Atlanta, Georgia) Journal*, March 3, 1987.

[6]Viegle, A. "If AIDS Question Not Answered Life Insurance Coverage Refused," *(New Orleans, Louisiana) Times-Picayune*, March 3, 1987.

[7]Viegle.

[8]Viegle.

[9]Viegle.

[10]Chambers 20.

[11]"Life Insurance in Force", *The 1986 Information Please Almanac* (New York: Houghton Mifflin Company) 48.

[12]Viegle.

[13]Buckley, W. F. "The AIDS Battle Needs More Than Alarm Ringing," *Molinee (Illinois) Daily Dispatch*, April 23, 1987: 4.

[14]Chambers 20.

[15]Price, J. "Medicaid Cuts in New Budget Seen Harming AIDS Patients," *Washington Times*, Jan. 12, 1987.

[16]Chapman, F. S. "AIDS & Business: Problems of Costs and Compassion," *Fortune*, Sept. 15, 1986: 127.

[17]Chapman 126.

[18]"Actuaries" 6.

[19]Chapman 127.

The Impact of AIDS on the Social Welfare System

The AIDS epidemic can potentially, and likely will, drastically change the social welfare system. According to current projections, productivity lost because of illness and premature deaths caused by AIDS could cost U.S. industry more than $55 billion in 1991. This may be an indication of the degree of stress to be placed on the social welfare system as AIDS decreases employment. It has been estimated that each AIDS patient now costs the American taxpayer between $150,000 and $300,000.

Token Efforts For Education

The U.S. Department of Health and Human Services recently awarded $15 million in grants to state and local governments to develop AIDS education programs for groups such as heterosexuals who are increasingly at risk of contracting the disease. Yet in England, where reported AIDS cases are one-quarter that of Canada (which is a fraction of U.S. cases), there is a full-scale public health crisis alert and a $40-million campaign to inform the public about AIDS, and *The Lancet* has suggested that Britain will have only 3,000 diagnosed cases of AIDS in 1988.

Certainly funding for public education is critically important. The frightening potential impact on the nation's social security "safety net," given continued sustained growth of AIDS, appears a vivid argument for drastic and immediate increase in public education funding. Among the subcomponents of the social welfare system ("safety net") which could be particularly affected by a massive increase in numbers of infected individuals are Medicare/Medicaid, Social Security Disability, Supplemental Security Income, and Unemployment Compensation.

Minority Groups and Children

Although it is true that AIDS is no respecter of position, it appears that some members of the lower socio-economic class may be particularly affected by the AIDS epidemic. Black and Hispanic women are up to 15 times more likely to become infected than white women. And women within the AIDS underclass are also the mothers of about 70% of the children who have contracted the disease. By 1991 some 3,000 children may have it—an eightfold increase from 1986. Those statistics bear a striking resemblance to the incidence of AIDS in central Africa, where the annual rate of infection is one adult in 1,000. Projecting the potential number of children infected by 2001, a number of 100,000 is not beyond reason, with a sizeable percentage from lower socio-economic groups.

Already children are being called the "third wave" of AIDS victims. "On any single day at Bellevue Hospital Center in downtown Manhattan, six babies and young children are being treated for [AIDS and] in nearby Newark, New Jersey, about 15 percent of the pediatric beds at Children's Hospital of New Jersey are occupied at any one time by youngsters with Acquired Immune Deficiency Syndrome."[1] Dr. Martha Rogers of CDC, who tracks AIDS's invasion of the national child population, has remarked, "The pediatric AIDS problem is a ticking time bomb [and] children are one of the fastest growing groups of AIDS patients in the United States." The Institute of Medicine of the U.S. National Academy of Sciences has stated that, for Africa, "possibly tens to hundreds of thousands of infants in Africa will die of AIDS in the next decade."[2] Could this be a harbinger of worse things to come in the United States?

The CDC now estimates that by the year 1991, more than 12,000 [American] children will have been diagnosed as having AIDS or ARC and that "it is quite possible that in certain major urban areas in the country, AIDS will kill more children than any other infectious disease."[3] Without doubt, children will be especially victimized by the disease.

Child welfare services for children from an AIDS-related family disruption may face difficulties. Dr. Andre Nahamies, professor of pediatrics at Emory University School of Medicine, stated that if a child is infected with the virus, it is almost a death sentence, because the child has about a 95 percent chance of developing AIDS and dying from it. As a result, "foster care placement may or may not be a problem. If the child is in a foster home when the diagnosis is made, these families may already have bonded with the child and will want to continue to care for him/her. For the child diagnosed before foster placement, however, the picture is more grim. Placement of these children remains difficult at best,"[4] and they may spend their short lives in a hospital-based care facility.

William Blacklow, an aide to Rep. George Miller (D-California) and chairman of a February 21, 1987 hearing in Berkeley, California of the House Select Committee on Children, Youth and Families, said about children born with AIDS, "We are inadequately prepared to take care of those babies who already have AIDS, let alone the many more who are likely to contract it in the near future. These children are on the border in every respect. They're neither here nor there in terms of care. Foster parents don't want to adopt them, the mother in some instances will not keep the baby and, because it's tremendously expensive, the hospitals can't afford to treat them. AIDS threatens to kill thousands of children."[5]

Directors of child care agencies often report "that children of AIDS patients [even if they themselves had no signs of the disease] could be placed only in homes with no other children,"[6] provided that those foster care homes can be located. Long-term placement (over 5 years) of children with AIDS has not been documented since "81% of children who were diagnosed with AIDS more than two years ago have died"[7] suffering from deadly forms of pneumonia, enlarged lymph nodes, infected blood, meningitis, strep, staph, salmonella, and urinary and ear infections as well as infections of the central nervous system, heart, liver and kidneys. Further, Jean McIntosh, assistant director of the Los Angeles County Department of Children's Services, has pointed out that fear of AIDS is "slowing the adoption and foster care of healthy babies because people are unwilling to take children of mothers who are intravenous drug users or members of other risk groups."[8]

Without doubt, as the numbers of adults who die and of infected children increase, children will be increasingly subject to discrimination and disruptions. Health officials are not optimistic about curbing the rate of pediatric AIDS because the women who are spreading it to their children tend to be drug users or associated with drug users and are outside the mainstream of health education. Perhaps predictive of a disturbing trend, there are reports that children born with AIDS may be among the experimental groups for preliminary vaccine/treatment—serving as society's guinea pigs.

Social Welfare Programming Needs and the Impact of AIDS

Other social welfare programs which will be required and which are used in some areas now include visiting nurses, home health services, homemaker care, psychological and social counseling, transportation services, buddy programs for AIDS victims, hot lines, nursing home services, hospice care, residential care, and foster care. Most of the costs for these programs will require federal assistance, straining the federal budget, or, if financed by state governments, will result in a tremendous increase in state taxes.

The current Medicare system (generally reserved only for those receiving social security benefits or, through state Medicaid programs, the financially indigent) pays approximately 80% of a patient's health care costs,[9] each Medicare/Medicaid—financed AIDS patient may need to contribute $9,800 per year (assuming the health care costs are $49,000 per person) or perhaps much more from some source towards their own care—an amount likely to quickly exhaust a victim's savings. More alarming, (Medicare/ Medicaid) hospital insurance does not pay the full cost of an in-patient stay in a skilled nursing facility, suggesting that, in reality, for the lower socio-economic class, the option of 24-hour-a-day skilled treatment may, under the current system, be impossible. The potential result of this economically-based health care discrimination may be that large numbers of the lower class receive essentially no treatment or substandard-treatment. Because of that, there will be increasing numbers of homeless, destitute persons and neglected children. As the numbers of homeless increase, the nation's crime rate can be expected to increase.

Stephen Smith, chairman of the Metropolitan Washington Committee on AIDS Issues, stated, "Medicaid is critical for AIDS patients. Without jobs and insurance, they have no alternative, unless they have a large amount of savings . . . So very large numbers of them—possibly even a majority —are forced to rely on Medical Assistance." Dr. Donald MacDonald of the Department of Health and Human Services said, the "Medicaid costs for AIDS patients was about $400 million in fiscal 1987"—this amount is only a beginning as AIDS cases skyrocket.[10] Suggesting even further stresses on Medicaid, G. H. Jones in *The Lancet* reports a case of "a 27-year old man known to have antibodies to HIV but who was otherwise healthy [whose] presumptive diagnosis was acute schizophrenia." Jones continued, "Could there be a link between this man's acute schizophrenic illness and his HIV carrier status, without symptoms of AIDS?"[11] If so, particularly when examined in light of the fact that AIDS attacks brain glia cells directly, Medicare/Medicaid funds may be even more greatly drained by psychiatric cases.

Nationalized Health Insurance?

Whether the Federal government will move to a nationalized health care system is debatable. Considering that in 1982, the Federal government spent $15.07 billion on health and medical care programs and 51% of the total federal budget outlays were for social welfare, it is unlikely that a nationalized health care system could be afforded without substantial reprioritization or increases in the federal budget. Assuming a minimum per-patient health care expense of $49,000 per year and only 1.5 million persons infected, a nationalized health care program which would *only* support AIDS patients would be 4.8 times the health and medical care programs expense of 1982 and a 20.05% increase in total federal outlays for social welfare (based on 1982 federal budget figures). Such tremendous additional costs in health and social welfare (and that only for health care for AIDS victims), particularly in light of the national debt, deficit, and national defense priorities, are not likely to be well received by a conservative congress.

AIDS and Other Social Security Programs

Certainly social security programs will be greatly strained through disbursal of benefits. Total family survivor benefits are estimated to be as high as $1,633 a month (per family) if the worker (died) in 1985. If *only* half of the A.D. 2001 estimated potential AIDS deceaseds' families are eligible for survivor benefits, and if only $800 a month per family is awarded, then *during the year 2001*, survivor benefits could approximate $7.2 billion. This amount is only a portion of the potential social security outlays.

Disability benefits will also put stress on the social security system. Monthly benefits in January 1985 or later can be as high as $909 for a worker and as high as $1,363 for a worker with a family. Once a person starts receiving benefits, the amount will increase automatically in future years to keep pace with the rising cost of living. Further, one may continue to receive disability benefits for up to 12 months after employment, even though the work is substantial, gainful work. If *only* half of the A.D. 2001 estimated potential AIDS-infected persons are eligible for disability benefits, and if *only* $700 a month per individual or family is awarded, then during the single year 2001 disability benefits could approximate $6.3 billion. Subtotal additional expenditures of social security outlays, including survivor benefits and disability, in A.D. 2001 *only* may approach $13.5 billion.

In 1986 supplemental security income payments of up to $325 a month for an individual and up to $488 for a couple can be made and States may supplement the federal payments. If *only* 25% of the A.D. 2001 estimated potential AIDS-infected persons are eligible for supplemental security income benefits, and if *only* $150 a month per individual or family is awarded, then, during the single year 2001, disability benefits could approximate $6.75 billion. Potential subtotal expenditure for just the year A.D. 2001 may be $20.25 billion. This amount combined with Medicare/Medicaid costs (discussed above) could push *yearly* social security program expenditures by 2001 to somewhere between $90-160 billion in additional costs over their mid-1980's level—an approximate increase of 40-75% in annual federal social welfare outlays (compared to mid-1980's funding). Total costs in A.D. 2001 for AIDS patient care for taxpayers may approach $450 billion or a 250% increase in expenditures. Projections for social security outlays in the out-years (2010) become much more grim—perhaps five times as much. This tremendous potential increase in social security outlays, a long-term consequence of failed planning now, could lead to the demise of that entire federal system.

AIDS and Unemployment Compensation

Mississippi has the lowest weekly unemployment compensation ($115) of any of the United States, with a maximum duration of benefits not to exceed 26 weeks. Assuming that only

10% of the projected 2001 AIDS cases become eligible for unemployment compensation and assuming that weekly benefits are $115 and that each case only maintains eligibility for 26 weeks (an across-all-States standard), the total unemployment compensation disbursed across the United States could approach $448.5 million during that year (2001) alone. This is a very conservative estimate. Further, as AIDS cases (in 1987) appear to be proportionately overdistributed in New York, California, Florida, Texas, New Jersey and Illinois, these states may be especially stressed. So far, 39% of AIDS cases in the U.S. have been in New York and San Francisco.

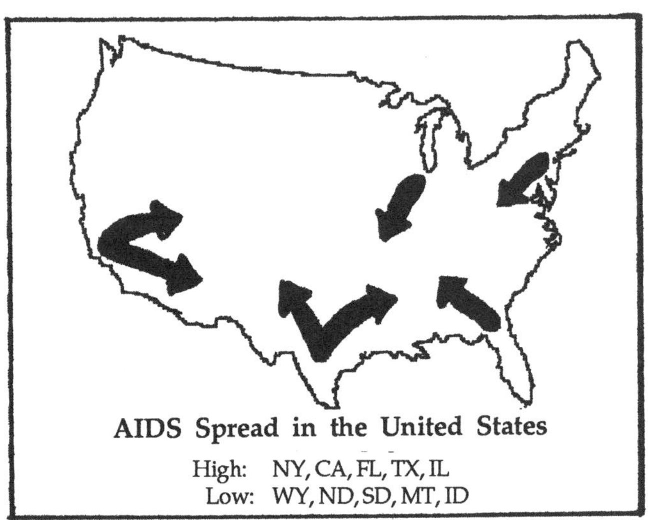

AIDS Spread in the United States

High: NY, CA, FL, TX, IL
Low: WY, ND, SD, MT, ID

Of interest from legal and economic viewpoints is the fact that already 21 states and several cities have legislation or court rulings that make AIDS a "protected handicap," a distinction that prohibits employers from firing people simply for having the disease. The degree to which this legislation is based on civil rights as compared to cost of AIDS-related unemployment, as these both relate to public health, is an interesting dilemma. It is not surprising that as the perceived risk of AIDS transfection remains low, the civil rights of AIDS victims remain paramout —the possibility of an economically-based bias toward de-emphasizing transfection risk through overemphasis of civil rights appears likely. Economists may err on a side detrimental to public health. More study of this potential is certainly necessary. Economics, without further study, should not be the major priority of any policy developments.

Epilogue

Efforts now in progress to forestall a major strain on the nation's social welfare system can be assessed in the strict upholding of AIDS victims' civil rights. To what extent civil rights rulings will allow continued employment of AIDS victims at the perceived risk to public health shall, in the long term, determine AIDS's impact on the social welfare system. When a "critical mass" of victims accrues in the United States, politics may outweigh economics. At that time, the exponential increase of AIDS-infected individuals may financially stress the social welfare system so much that they will be denied continued employment.

Modest projections for annual social welfare system costs for A.D. 2001 suggest an increase of some 10-20% above those of the mid-1980's—equivalent to a $30-60 billion dollar annual increase in federal social welfare expenditures over 1984 levels. Some states may be severely challenged to provide unemployment compensation as the number of AIDS cases rises and may seek federal help at a time when the federal budget is under great stress.

These "safety net" services, increasing in annual cost at a time when the federal and most states' budgets may show a deficit, suggest the possibility of drastic change in the type and manner of social welfare service delivery. Not unlikely, under extreme grassroot political pressure, a "not affordable" national health insurance system will be enacted, perhaps based on an expanded version of Medicare. Those funds, in a "rob Peter to pay Paul" strategy, will likely be drawn from other social security funds. At the same time, there may be increased disbursals from those other funds (e.g., social security retirement, survivor benefits, disability, and supplemental security income accounts).

This temporary "line item transfer," a simplistic short-term solution, will quickly be found incapable of disbursing the required outlays, necessitating a reprioritization of federal funding, an increase in social security taxes, an increase in the national debt, or a reduction of benefits in other than the most basic AIDS care-related services. This strategy, if forced by grass-root political pressure, will likely result in an increased number of "fixed-income" persons receiving greatly reduced support: the old, survivors of AIDS-deceased parents, the disabled, the unemployed. The social welfare system may, of necessity, be forced to return to charity systems such as existed before 1933.

The most prudent planning to facilitate a minimum down-grading of social welfare services appears to be that which is based on maintenance of AIDS-victims' civil rights and based on creation of minimally state/federal supported community-based programs. This planning, in anticipation of grassroot political pressures to abandon AIDS-victims' civil rights, must certainly be in progress by 1989 and "on-line" in the early '90s.

Notes

[1]Seabrook, C. "AIDS in Kids 'A Ticking Time Bomb,'" *(Atlanta) Georgia Journal*, Feb. 19, 1987.

[2]Seabrook.

[3]Kotulak, R. "AIDS Cases Increasing Among Kids," *Chicago Tribune*, Feb. 1, 1987.

[4]Klug, R. M. "Children With AIDS," *American Journal of Nursing*, Oct. 1986:1132.

[5]Barnhill, M. "AIDS Slows Adoptions of Babies," *(Los Angeles, California) Daily News*, Feb. 23, 1987.

[6]Brosnan, S. "Our First Home Care AIDS Patient: Maria," *Nursing86*, Sept. 1986: 39.

[7]Klug 1126.

[8]Barnhill.

[9]"Medicare Program"; *The 1986 Information Please Almanac* (Houghton Mifflin Company, 60 East 42 Street, New York, NY) 334.

[10]Price, J. "Medicaid Cuts in New Budget Seen Harming AIDS Patients," *Washington Times*, Jan. 12, 1987.

[11]Jones, G. H., et al. "HIV and Onset of Schizophrenia," *The Lancet*, April 25, 1987: 982.

The Impact of AIDS on the Federal Government System

> "Prince Prospero was happy and dauntless and sagacious. When his dominions were half depopulated, he summoned to his presence a thousand hale and light-hearted friends from among the knights and dames of his court, and with these retired to the deep seclusion of one of his castellated abbeys. This was an extensive and magnificient structure, the creation of the prince's own eccentric yet august taste. A strong and lofty wall girdled it in. This wall had gates of iron. The courtiers, having entered, brought furnaces and massy hammers and welded the bolts. They resolved to leave means neither of ingress or egress to the sudden impulses of despair or of frenzy from within. The abbey was amply provisioned. With such precautions the courtiers might bid defiance to contagion. The external world could take care of itself. In the meantime it was folly to grieve, or to think. The prince had provided all the appliances of pleasure. There were buffoons, there were improvisatori, there were ballet-dancers, there were musicians, there was Beauty, there was wine. All these and security were within. Without was the 'Red Death.'
>
> *The Masque of the Red Death,* by Edgar Allen Poe

Citing Canadian government policy on AIDS, Barbara Amiel stated, "Returning to Canada [from England and comparing national AIDS strategies] is like going through the looking glass backward. Canada is next door to the United States, the major center of AIDS in the Western world. But what is this country [Canada] doing about it? It is true that Canadian doctors have been holding conferences and trying to alert public awareness, *but government policy on the matter is close to the bizarre.*"[1] If Canadian governmental policy is "bizarre" what then can be said about the U. S. government's policy? "If silence remains the response of national leaders to a special hell awaiting U. S. young people and their families, then those leaders will no longer have any credibility to discuss moral values or to profess their concern for youth."[2]

The Government Was Caught Off Guard

Gary McDonald, executive director of the AIDS Action Council of the Federation of AIDS-Related Organizations in Washington, D. C., stated, "It's obvious that the [U. S.] government was caught off guard and is still off guard. The federal government in general—and the Public Health Service in particular—is not equipped to respond to such a devastating epidemic."[3] Ann Fettner, author of *The Truth About AIDS*, has remarked, "Federal agencies have been forceful in leading efforts in prevention, screening, and treatment of other diseases, yet they have done very little with respect to AIDS. The government has done literally nothing in the way of education"[4] and education is currently the only means advocated of preventing the spread of the disease. In January 1987, Dr. Mervyn F. Silverman, president of the American Foundation for AIDS Research, said, "We have no national policy for AIDS and I think that is a disgrace. We are seeing very little money put into education, which is our only defense at this time. We're seeing very little money put into care."[5]

Lack of Presidential Leadership

Dr. David Baltimore, Nobel Prize-winning biologist, has remarked, "We [the scientific community] are quite honestly frightened about the prospects here and feel [that the problem] requires Presidential leadership."[6] The President, making his first public statements about AIDS during early April 1987, responded with "it's not how you do it—it's don't do it." During March 1987, the Reagan administration, after months of internal dispute, finally agreed to approve an aggressive AIDS education effort only if that education emphasizes sexuality within the context of marriage and teaches children to avoid sex. During May 1987, the President announced formation of a national commission to advise him on ways of dealing with the spread of AIDS. The commission will review research, assess the long-term impact on the health-care system, and recommend ways to protect those who do not have the disease, but the commission will have only advisory powers and will not be separate from already existing cabinet offices. It appears that the administration is still not reacting as forcefully as is necessary to the crisis.

Specifically, the administration's support for AIDS education efforts are based on these principles:

1. Any health information developed under federal government auspices or by the federal government directly should encourage responsible sexual behavior based on fidelity, commitment and maturity, placing sexuality within the context of marriage.

2. Educational material to be used in schools should teach that children should not engage in sex and that any educational material should be used only with the consent and involvement of parents.

3. The federal government should not mandate specific school courses or curriculum for AIDS education, but should trust the American people to use this educational information in a manner appropriate to their community's needs.

Other than requesting a report from the Surgeon General, an April 1987 Presidential statement encouraging abstinance as a way to reduce risk and establishing an advisory committee, the White House has been absolutely quiet on the issue of AIDS. Secretary of Education William Bennett told textbook writers only that he expects curriculum materials on AIDS to become a growth industry. Despite the administration's desire to emphasize restraint in sex as a way to check the spread of the disease, direct leadership is not forthcoming.

More Educational Funding Is Necessary

The Department of Health and Human Services has awarded subcontracts to develop some AIDS education initiatives, but the amount provided for education appears minimal when compared to that of Great Britain. The ratio of U. S. to British AIDS cases is approximately 52 to 1 (based on September 19, 1986 World Health Organization and Centers for Disease Control data), yet current British AIDS education support is $40 million—approximately 20 percent of the United States expenditures. The total U. S. federal budget for AIDS was approximately $400 million in 1986, half of which went for education and half for vaccine development, and only 10 times that of Britain's 1986

AIDS educational programming. The U. S. federal government proposed to spend a total of approximately $500 million on AIDS during fiscal 1988, including $150 million for education and prevention. At the same time, the National Academy of Sciences recommended quadrupling Federal funding for AIDS research and education to $2 billion. To be comparable to Great Britain's effort of AIDS funding-per-citizen, the National Academy of Sciences figure is appropriate.

Federal Funding for the AIDS Battle and Medicare/Medicaid

"Every year since 1984, the White House has proposed spending less on AIDS programs than the Public Health Service wanted to, and much less than Congress eventually appropriated. The $411 million AIDS budget for 1987 was almost double the administration's proposal. For fiscal year 1988, the administration proposes to hike AIDS spending to $534 million, a nod to increasing public health concerns but still far less than many experts recommend."[7] Yet President Reagan has proposed $6 billion in cuts for Medicare and Medicaid in 1988. Dr. Massimo Righini, chairman of the board of the D. C. Medical Society, said, "We know many AIDS patients are winding up in Medicaid and welfare programs because they become unemployed as a result of their disease and exhaust their savings,"[8] yet the administration proposed a $25.4 billion cap on federal Medical Assistance payments in fiscal 1988. The trend to limit Medicare/Medicaid funding in light of the increasing reliance of AIDS victims on this support may create problems ahead.

Administration Irresponsibility?

With social security outlays potentially approaching $30-60 billion for AIDS-related benefits alone as early as 2001 and statements by the Surgeon General that a vaccine may not be available until that time, it appears that the federal government is not acting responsibly to forestall a potential disaster. Most health officials believe the Federal Government will have to take a larger role not only in education but in other areas if an AIDS disaster is to be avoided. The Reagan administration, like most Americans, is betting on a scientific breakthrough to deliver America from the epidemic, yet it is unlikely that this will occur and the consequence of a lost wager will be catastrophic.

A recent report by the National Institute of Medicine and the National Academy of Sciences states that "efforts to combat AIDS will require at least $2 billion a year by 1990, more than five times the present level of expenditure. About half the funds should be spent on research, but perhaps the most pressing need is to put more resources into explicit and extensive education programs."[9] This call-to-arms has identified a lack of cohesiveness and strategic planning throughout the nation as a major source of concern, and the report's main message, according to Dr. Sheldon Wolff, chairman of the department of medicine at Tufts University School of Medicine, is that AIDS isn't something confined to a subpopulation. It's a very serious problem for the whole community.[10] This report warns that disease and death are likely to be increasing 5 to 10 years from now and probably into the next century and that a massive, coordinated campaign to educate the general public is critical. It also warns that if government agencies continue to be unable or unwilling to use direct, explicit terms in the detailed content of educational programs, contractual arrangements should be established with private organizations that are not subject to the same inhibitions.

The Surgeon General's Efforts

Certainly, of all federal government administration officials to date, Surgeon General C. Everett Koop has surfaced as a leader, though reluctantly, in the battle against AIDS. *US News and World Report* stated that "Koop's outspokenness is being applauded—this recent [Surgeon General's Report on AIDS] report went straight to the point in explicit language [and] was a breakthrough for a federal document."[11] Though AIDS has finally become "real" and, as of April 6, 1987, become the nation's number one health concern (over cancer and health care costs)—it has had such a head start that the federal government must act quickly and assert itself as a leader, follow Europe's educational models, or face the potential of an AIDS panic.

A Possible Scenario?

Given the Federal Government's current lack of leadership, apparent insufficient funding, and failure to realistically plan for the future, the following scenario may not be unrealistic:

> It is the year 2001: the number of AIDS-diagnosed persons is 3.5 million. 1.5 million persons will die this year and 50 million may be infected but not yet diagnosed. After several short-term shifts in social security funds, it is now apparent that the system may be near collapse. Survivor and Disability benefits have been slashed and Medicare, hastily nationalized in the mid 1990's, threatens to gobble up 20-50% of yearly social welfare expenditures.
>
> A large number of destitute and homeless concentrate in certain cities and the crime rates in those areas rises dramatically. Anarchy is imminent. As a result of reprioritization, while maintaining a committment to national defense, and meeting the national health care emergency, the annual Federal fiscal budget now approaches $5 trillion—the annual budget deficit $1 trillion—the Federal debt $10 trillion.
>
> Of necessity, the President has declared a national emergency suspending civil liberties. The military, in some areas, is assisting in providing both patient care and martial law. A major devaluation of the currency, resulting from inability to control a run-away budget, imminently threatens the economic security of the nation. The U.S., as a sovereign nation based on individual freedom, is on the verge of collapse.

Again science fiction? James Miller, director of the Office of Management and Budget, worries that in 20 years, a significant portion of our society could be incapacitated and we could end up with two societies—those that have it (AIDS) and those that don't. Conservative estimates put the number of victims of AIDS worldwide at 100 million by 1990. The U.S., where the most comprehensive records are kept, has the highest number of reported cases of any nation in the world, other than central African nations, as of September 1986. If only 10% of those cases projected for 1990 are in the U.S., by the year 2001 the effect of AIDS on the nation could be devastating. The number of U.S. AIDS cases may be 3-4 million diagnosed with, perhaps, 50 million infected but not yet diagnosed in 2001. Such is the potential magnitude of this disease.

Epilogue

The Federal budget for AIDS has risen from $5.5 million to $411 million over the last five years and will rise to $534 million per year by 1988. In the fiscal year 1986, Federal outlay per AIDS victim was $16,108 based on 25,515 victims; the fiscal year 1988 Federal outlay per AIDS victim will be $7,240 based on 75,000 victims. The Federal funding ratio is, in fact, declining. By 1988 AIDS cases may approach 2.9 times the 1986 level while Federal funding may be only 44% of 1986 levels per victim. The 1988 level of funding will not keep pace with the growth of the disease nor will it likely keep pace with AIDS growth from now on. To maintain funding at the level of 1986 for AIDS-related interventions, the Federal Government outlay in 1988 must be $1.2 *billion*. By 1995 perhaps $50 billion will be necessary.

The degree of federal leadership to date, especially Presidential leadership, when compared to the European and Japanese response, has been abominable. The absence of aggressive leadership and long-term planning, based on a notion that a scientific breakthrough will occur, appears a major gamble, as the likelihood of a timely vaccine and potential risk are considered. The results of a lost wager, which could destroy the social fabric of the nation, appear too great a risk. AIDS will pose profound questions to American society and test its reserves of compassion and common sense. Should AIDS in America in 2001 approach what is projected for Africa, one in every two sexually active adults will be infected.

If the Federal Government does not *now* begin to take the epidemic extremely seriously, it is not beyond reason to expect that, by the year 2001, AIDS will have pushed the U.S. into a corner. The massive drain on the Federal budget, from either existing or new health and/or welfare benefits, will leave the Government without many options. At the very least it is likely that Federal welfare systems will be drastically changed. What that change may be depends upon actions taken now.

In an almost bizarre occurrence (on May 31, 1987), Administration officials at an international AIDS conference in Washington, D.C., proposing manditory testing of selected subpopulations of the U.S., e.g., federal prisoners, were "booed" by some participants of the conference. Even with these modest proposals to approach disease containment, the administration has met resistance, suggesting that AIDS is to become an increasingly politicized issue.

Politicization of AIDS will surely reduce the ability of the federal government to effectively intervene in containing the disease.

The present course of Federal neglect of the "plague" and resistance to any modest federal disease-containment initiatives will probably result in a worse scenario: 1) Social security retirement benefits will cease. 2) Social security death benefits will cease. 3) Social security disability benefits will either cease or be drastically cut. 4) Social security survivor benefits will cease or be greatly curtailed. 5) Medicare/Medicaid budgets will be drained and economic ruin will loom. In short, the federal government could be greatly disrupted.

> "It was then, however, that the Prince Prospero, maddening with rage and the shame of his own momentary cowardice, rushed hurriedly through the six chambers, while none followed him on account of a deadly terror that had seized upon all. He bore aloft a drawn dagger, and had approached, in rapid impetuosity, to within three or four feet of the retreating figure, when the later, having attained the extremity of the velvet apartment, turned suddenly and confronted his pursuer. There was a sharp cry—and the dagger dropped gleaming upon the sable carpet, upon which, instantly afterwards, fell prostrate in death the Prince Prospero.
>
> And now was acknowledged the presence of the Red Death. He had come like a thief in the night. And one by one dropped the revellers in the blood-bedewed halls of their revel, and died each in the despairing posture of his fall. And the life of the ebony clock went out with that of the last of the gay. And the flames of the tripods expired. And Darkness and Decay and the Red Death held illimitable dominion over all."

The Masque of the Red Death, by Edgar Allen Poe

[1] Amiel, B. "The Politics of a Killer Disease"; *Maclean's*, Dec. 8, 1986: 11.

[2] Lewis, A. C. "A Dangerous Silence"; *Phi Delta Kappan*, Jan. 1987: 348.

[3] Lieberson, J. (moderator) "AIDS: What is to be Done?, *Harper's* Oct. 1985: 46.

[4] Lieberson 46.

[5] Smith, R. "AIDS Policy Called Too Little, Too Late," *Akron (Ohio) Beacon Journal*, Jan. 31, 1987.

[6] Lewis, A. C. "A Dangerous Silence"; *Phi Delta Kappan,* Jan. 1987: 348.

[7] McAuliffe, K., "AIDS: At the Dawn of Fear"; *U. S. News and World Report,* Jan. 12, 1987: 62.

[8] "More Funds Sought for AIDS Research; Health Plans Trimmed," *Washington (D. C.) Times,* Jan. 7, 1987.

[9] Norman, C. "$2-Billion Program Urged for AIDS," *Science* 234.4777: 661.

[10] Norman 661.

[11] McAuliffe 65.

The Impact of AIDS on the Legal/Constitutional System

"Our social values seem at least as firmly bound to money as they were at the turn of the century; in developing the biological methods needed to prevent disease, we face growing propensities to sue for damages in the absence of a national health system and other social supports and protection."[1] As a result of the AIDS epidemic, interesting legal and constitutional issues appear to be occurring now and promise to escalate as the disease spreads. Areas receiving attention now are those which involve discrimination and violation of Article 4 of the Amendments to the U. S. Constitution.

Employee HTLV-III/LAV Testing

Testing prospective employees to determine if they have antibodies against the AIDS virus has been used by some employers and is extremely controversial. Proposals to require such antibody tests as a public health measure were quashed at a meeting held by the Centers for Disease Control in early March 1987. Reasons for arguing against pre-employment blood testing for AIDS may be many, but could potentially rest on Article 4 of the amendments to the U.S. Constitution (*Bill of Rights*): "The right of the people to be secure in their person, houses, papers, and effects, against unreasonable searches and seizures, shall not be violated, and no warrants shall issue, but upon probable cause, supported by oath or affirmation, and particularly describ-ing the place to be searched, and the persons or things to be seized."

Despite CDC's stand against testing prospective employees for antibodies, some companies are using the blood tests. Dallas-based Ensearch Corp. screens food-service employees, even though a spokesman admits there is no medical evidence that AIDS can be transmitted through food or casual contact. Some experts charge that companies are surreptitiously testing employee's blood samples that were taken for other reasons. Others believe some employers are illegally using such common employment application questions as "Are you married?" in an attempt to screen out potential AIDS patients.[2]

Employees Refusing to Work With the AIDS Infected

Legal questions regarding employees with AIDS or other employees refusing to work with an employee with AIDS appear confusing. Irwin Davison, attorney for the New York City Department of Public Health, has pointed out that an employer may have little legal choice but to strongly discipline workers who refuse to work with an AIDS victim. He remarked, "Failure to take such a strong action may put the company at risk for a successful chance of employment discrimination."[3]

Alternatively, Judge Benjamin Nolan, an administrator of the New York City Civil Court, suggested in 1985 that an employee would have a cause of action for money damages against an employer if the employer caused an employee to acquire AIDS by ordering the employee to work with an AIDS victim without allowing the employee to wear protective garb.[4] In 1986 employees afraid of working with an AIDS victim had some legal protection under two federal statutes. The Occupational Safety and Health Administration requires that workplaces be free of recognized hazards and the National Labor Relations Act requires that employees cannot be penalized for refusing to work out of legitimate fear for their safety. Of note, the OSHA act was struck down—it is not a legal option; the NLR Act has not yet been tested.

To further confuse the picture, in 1986 the Justice Department issued an opinion that the provision forbidding discrimination against the handicapped does not apply to AIDS victims if the employer is motivated by fear that the disease may spread. Thus an employer who fired an AIDS victim would be exempt from prosecution under federal statute *if* the firing was based on a perceived danger that other employees were in danger of contracting AIDS.

On March 3, 1987, however, the Supreme Court ruling in *School Board of Nassau County vs. Arline,* a case where a teacher who was fired because of tuberculosis was reinstated and the disease considered "a handicap" under Section 504 of the Rehabilitation Act of 1973. This Section prohibits discrimination against the handicapped and seems to have effectively negated the Justice Department's 1986 decision although it prohibits handicap discrimination by recipients of federal funds only.

Even though this Supreme Court precedential ruling has been decreed regarding disease and handicap and receipt of federal funding, there has not yet been a case before the Supreme Court testing AIDS directly. It is unknown how the Court might rule on the issue. The critical point may rest on whether AIDS is ruled contagious —a potentially inflammatory decision.

Testing Potential Insurees

Testing prospective insurees for HTLV-III/LAV has provoked additional complaints of discrimination whether that testing is based on blood-antibody presence or based on questions designed to detect AIDS high-risk group membership. Great Republic Insurance Company, of Santa Barbara, California asked single men such questions as whether they were antique dealers, interior decorators, consultants, and florists (apparently presumed by Great Republic to be occupations with high percentages of homosexuals) and was subsequently taken to court on discrimination charges.

To prevent the possibility of discrimination based on blood testing, some cities and states have banned (antibody) testing. As a result, some insurance companies are not marketing their services in those regions. For more information regarding this area, see the chapter entitled *The Impact of Aids on Insurance.*

Other Legal Questions

Other AIDS-related legal actions occurring include damage suits brought against hospitals, doctors, and blood banks from which persons contracted AIDS through transfusion. It appears likely that these cases may be won by plantiffs. Lawrence Gostin, an attorney at the Harvard School of Public Health and director of the American Society of Legal Medicine stated in 1987, "For the first time we are seeing how inadequate the law can be in dealing with public health matters . . . the inadequacies of public health law—not just with AIDS but with many other diseases."[4]

Attorney Alex M. Clarke of the American Bar Association's committee on health law stated in 1987, "At this point, the law growing around AIDS has nothing to do with public health law. It has something to do with the protection of the individual—not safeguarding the public health."[5] Gostin also points out the dilemma facing the public health system relating to developing law, saying that health officials are being forced to rely on education and voluntary screening programs to limit the epidemic. Compulsory programs would simply drive people who might transmit AIDS underground and destroy the confidence public health officials need to get their cooperation. Lack of compulsory programs in public health law does, however, drive AIDS cases to the civil and criminal courts where cases revolve around the rights of individuals.

It can be argued with some success that in avoiding establishing compulsory programming the public health network is allowing, by default, public health law to be written by the civil courts where individual rights may supercede the rights of the collective. Realistically, do we know enough about AIDS to allow public health law to be written by non-experts?

Legal Questions in the Future

In the future a legal "heyday" may be in the making as AIDS cases continue to increase. Among the potential legal issues which may be tested in the courts are:

1. Can damages be awarded to an employee from an employer if the employee becomes infected and is not of a high risk group, does not engage in high risk behavior, and has had contact with an AIDS victim only at the job site?

2. Can a parent be awarded damages from an educational institution if the child develops AIDS and is not of a high risk group, does not engage in high risk behavior, and has had contact with an AIDS victim only at the school site?

3. Can a parent be awarded damages from a private preschool/daycare facility if the child develops AIDS and has had no other

source of contact if, through blood testing, it is found that another child is infected—even if the preschool/daycare facility was not aware of the infected child's status?

4. Can an AIDS victim sue the person from whom they contracted the disease if it is proved that that other person was the only source of disease contact?

5. Will the National Labor Relations Act allow employees to band together to force an employer to terminate an infected employee?

6. Can schools be sued by parents for not providing adequate educational information to students in those cases where a student develops AIDS?

7. Can local/state/regional Public Health Departments be sued by AIDS victims for improper or insufficient public education regarding the disease?

8. Can insurance companies be sued for releasing an insurees blood-test results to medical information bureaus?

9. Can a class action suit of reverse discrimination be filed by employees in a firm where an AIDS victim is employed?

10. Can an AIDS patient sue a hospital in cases where it has been proven discriminatory health care practices have occurred, e.g., improper mouth care for oral thrush?

11. Can an AIDS patient file a malpractice suit against his doctor as a result of improper treatment or failure to provide "state-of-the art" treatment?

12. Can a tenant, who becomes infected by the AIDS virus, sue his/her landlord claiming the virus was transmitted from the residence?

13. What are the legal liabilities of a corporation whose employee, suffering from AIDS dementia, causes a major loss of life through negligence?

14. Will the Supreme Court rule that AIDS is a contagious disease and will the disease be considered a handicap?

These questions and countless others will be tested as the AIDS epidemic continues. Although legal precedential analogues may exist, because of this uniquely deadly retrovirus's potential and the rapidity of scientific information change, much new legal ground will be broken in the near future.

AIDS and the Constitution

From a constitutional standpoint, an extremely interesting vote occurred in California during November 1986. Ballot Proposition 64 was designed to legally declare AIDS as an "infectious, contagious, and easily communicable disease." It would have "forced public health officials to establish camps to quarantine AIDS patients and anyone who carries the AIDS virus, and flatly ban persons infected by the virus from attending or teaching in public schools or holding jobs that involve food handling. The proposition was placed for vote before the general population and defeated 2 to 1.

Disconcerting because of its potential assault on constitutional freedoms, the organization Prevent AIDS Now Initiative California (PANIC) had no trouble getting 683,000 California voters to sign the petition that put Proposition 64 on the ballot. Furthermore, Proposition 64, associated with the Lyndon LaRouche Organization and explained in a LaRouche-published magazine *Executive Intelligence Review*, was defeated in California, but as the epidemic increases and substantial federal guid-ance fails to materialize, may likely appear in other forms in other states.

Quarantine as a method of containing the disease, according to James Mason, head of the CDC and acting assistant secretary for health, has been discussed by federal officials. Public health deans, in arguing against a quarantine approach in California (Proposition 64), concluded that Proposition 64 would throw 36,000 people out of work needlessly, and would cost $1.2 billion per year just to test the education and food-handling population for AIDS antibodies. The cost of internment of a large population in quarantine is not known. Quarantine might have stopped the disease in its early days. Now it would face insuperable hurdles—where to put the millions who have the virus, and what they are to do for the rest of their lives, which can be respectably long.[6]

Would quarantine and massive blood-testing of the population be happening now if it didn't cost billions of dollars? It is a logical question. If that were possible, then a logical deduction seems to be that economics is a major factor now protecting our civil liberties. At the same time, economics threaten longer-term survival. Ronald Bayer, co-director of the Hasting's Center Project on AIDS, has stated, "It's clear mass quarantine couldn't work, at least not in a way that would benefit public health; but it would have a profound effect on civil liberties."[7] Is Bayer suggesting that quarantine couldn't work because of prohibitive cost—and, if so, at what potential longer-term social costs?

State and Local AIDS Legislation

State and local-level anti-discriminatory legislation for AIDS victims is sparse, but the disease may constitute a handicap under states' disability and handicapped laws. The State of Florida, for example, on April 7, 1986 through the Florida Commission on Human Rights, affirmed that firing Broward County budget analyst Todd Shuttleworth, an AIDS victim, was unlawful. His subsequent lawsuit claimed $5 million in compensatory damages for lost pay, estimated fringe benefits, humiliation, and emotional distress. State and local litigation appears to be on the increase.

In 1986 more than 200 AIDS-related bills were introduced in 35 states, 160 of which were rejected or withdrawn. Some of these bills give an idea of what may be on the horizon. West Virginia heard a proposal to make the transmission of AIDS a first-degree-murder crime. A Colorado bill would have made AIDS transmission punishable by 4 years in prison. Hawaii would have made it a felony for an infected person to donate blood or put others at risk through sexual contact. Alabama would have quarantined—indefinitely—all prisoners with AIDS. Nan D. Hunter, of the ACLU in New York City, stated, "The threat of increased restrictive legislative proposals will worsen each year because the number of AIDS cases is increasing yearly. As the number of people affected directly or indirectly grows, so too will the perceived need to regulate more stringently."[8]

preceived need to regulate more stringently."[8]

Woodrow A. Meyers Jr., State Health Commissioner for Indiana, asked the Indiana General Assembly for authority to quarantine carriers of the AIDS virus who are sexually promiscuous and who have not taken steps to prevent transmission of the virus. So far, the Indiana General Assembly has not responded, but members of the Indiana Senate Health and Human Services Committee unanimously recommended passage of Senate Bill 72 which would allow "a county health officer to get a court order to restrict a person with a communicable disease, including AIDS . . . and restrictions could include isolation/quarantine if there is a showing of clear and convincing evidence of the serious and present health threat to others posed by the individual."[9] Further the Senate bill also outlines that a doctor, hospital or medical lab that fails to report confirmed cases of AIDS to the state health board could be charged with a class A infraction, carrying a $10,000 maximum fine as well as procedures for a student to be excluded from school. Indiana House Bill 1010, under discussion during February 1987, also would allow for isolating patients with communicable disease.

In California where efforts have been made to develop policies that would, as a last resort, place malicious and irresponsible AIDS-infected "spreaders" (e.g., a prostitute with AIDS who refuses to urge customers to use condoms) in isolation or quarantine, strenuous resistance has developed. Bruce Decker, chairman of the California AIDS advisory committee has argued that efforts to incorporate criminal sanctions against AIDS spreaders "threatens to turn public health clinics into centers for incrimination."[10] Keith Griffin, an AIDS activist in California, said regarding the proposal to incarcerate AIDS spreaders, "we will organize massive resistance on a scale that will disrupt everyone's existence in California—[proposals such as this may violate] people's civil rights in the name of public health."[11] Does an individual have the civil right to continue to pass a certain death sentence on an unsuspecting public? Aren't rights of any kind ultimately earned through the result of responsibility?

In Georgia, a bill giving health officials powers to require examination and treatment of people suffering from AIDS, to order tests for pregnant women and to force AIDS sufferers to divulge their sex partners was passed by the Georgia House. Already it appears that, because of early civil libertarian defense of individual rights, some state legislatures are attempting to pass legislation which, being backlash measures to that civil rights activity, may in the longer term erode civil liberties. Civil rights activists must, it appears, focus realistically on disease containment if their desire is truly the preservation of civil liberties.

In a different legal twist, Nurse Norma Watson, at San Francisco General Hospital, who complained "that working with AIDS patients gave her an ulcer" was awarded approximately $5,000 in temporary disability payments by the City of San Francisco. She alleged that her "supervisors orally instructed her that she had to treat AIDS patients ungloved and unmasked and that then she became ill with the ulcer and the stress."[12] California state Occupational Safety and Health Administration (OSHA) said in September 1985 that nurses had the right to wear protective clothing when working with AIDS patients, thus Nurse Watson complained to the state labor commission and subsequently settled out of court.

Epilogue

Because AIDS is a uniquely new disease, past legal precedents may not stand as the disease spreads in the future to the general population. Despite recent Supreme Court rulings to the contrary, the civil rights of AIDS patients will be increasingly challenged as the numbers of cases increase and the fears of the general population increase. This may be accomplished through state legislation of the California Proposition 64 variety. "As cases mount, how many 'liberal' values—the right to privacy and confidentiality, the civil rights won during the past decade or two by vulnerable minorities—might be eroded or even swept away by hysteria over AIDS?"[13]

It is not unlikely that an increasing number of damage suits will be filed against individuals and institutions, particularly in the absence of health and life insurance benefits for victims and the absence of a national health care system or a suitable community-based response. The seeds of potential prolific litigation appear to be evolving now through insurance companies' requirements for blood tests, governmental banning of blood tests as discriminatory in certain communities, and the responding action of insurance companies to cease coverage of those communities.

Challenges to Article 4 of the *Bill of Rights* may erode

freedom from personal searches, particularly if a blood test for AIDS becomes manditory. Challenges to Article 8 of the *Bill of Rights* may redefine rules regarding incarceration if quarantine for AIDS victims becomes mandatory. Other constitutional rights may be weakened or suspended and, with non-main-stream political groups' continued activity in seeking testing, labeling, and quarantine of AIDS victims, the frequency of these challenges may increase. It is not beyond possibility that erosion of constitutional freedoms will come not from the government but by demand from a frightened, uneducated population. The stage is now being set for a backlash of fear—caution is advised. Ronald Bayer, of the Hastings Center Project on AIDS asks, "How does one fashion a vigorous public health response while at the same time acknowledging the importance of protecting privacy and civil liberties?" And he answers, "Frankly, I don't be-lieve privacy and civil liberties are compatible with such a vigor-ous response. If we continue to claim that they are, we may find ourselves with policies that ignore civil liberties altogether."[14]

As the AIDS epidemic becomes increasingly litigated rather than being discussed in a true and rational way, the nation may be forced to place economic considerations above the practice of common sense and scientific observation. If economic considera-tions are foremost, as it seems now, the only winner in the end will be the disease. Rationality must be sustained. "The concern for privacy, civil liberties, and constitutional rights has become so pre-eminent in the past few decades that it is impossible to de-termine at what point these individual protections might be compromised in the name of public health."[15]

Notes

1 Yankauer, A. "The Persistence of Public Health Problems," *AJPH* 76. 5, May 1986: 495.

2 Chapman, F. S. "AIDS & Business: Problems of Costs and Compassion," *Fortune* Sept. 15, 1986: 127.

3 Stoller, B. "AIDS," *The Journal of Practical Nursing* Dec. 1985: 31.

[4] Sternberg, S. "AIDS Outbreak Spawns Growing Epidemic of Lawsuits," *Atlanta (Georgia) Journal,* Jan. 17, 1987.

[5] Sternberg.

[6] "A Plague on Everyone," *The Economist,* Nov. 22, 1986: 16.

[7] Lieberson, J. (moderator) "AIDS: What is to be Done?, *Harper's* Oct. 1985: 47.

[8] Lamb, D. "Colorado AIDS Bill Raises New Discrimination Fears," *Los Angeles (California) Times,* Jan. 26, 1987.

[9] Krause, R. A. "Law Would Allow Isolating AIDS Patients," *(Gary, Indiana Post-Tribune* Feb. 25, 1987.

[10] Brazil, E. "State Revising Proposal on AIDS Spreaders," *San Francisco (California) Examiner,* Feb. 26, 1987.

[11] Brazil.

[12] Fernandez, E. "Nurse Awarded $5,000 for Stress of Treating AIDS," *San Francisco (California) Examiner,* Feb. 20, 1987.

[13] Lieberson 50.

[14] Lieberson 51.

[15] Lieberson 47.

The Impact of AIDS on the Social Fabric of America

How AIDS will affect the social fabric of America can only be suggested. Its potential impact appears ominous. Consider the following scenario:

> It's the year 2001. Since 1995, the heterosexual community has seen a death rate comparable to that seen in the homosexual community in the late-1980s. The disease, now in A. D. 2001, is reported to have infected nearly 50 million persons in the United States and dire predictions of even higher rates in the near-term future have been made. A person's odds of contracting AIDS is now 1 out of 5 from sexual contacts. What is extremely unnerving is that the disease is prevalent in the very young adult and late-teens population. Finding a potential marriage partner is a frightening business. Some families, in anticipation of this very problem, have now arranged marriages for their children and the idea is gaining strength.
>
> Because of the massive numbers of persons sick or disabled from the disease, the nation's workforce is insufficient to meet the needs of many industries and services. Shortages of goods have become the rule of the day and families have, of necessity, become more self sufficient. This intrafamilial reliance has greatly strengthened the concept of the extended family and many families have 3 generations living together as a unit.
>
> Institutional health care costs have risen astronomically and, as a result, seeking medical help for relatively minor problems has ceased. Further, because of major budget cuts to federal social welfare programs some communities have developed health care collectives with minor care (minor is now defined as anything which does not require surgery) being provided by, what would in a less-developed society be called, shaman: older "wise" persons. This function, being filled by some older persons is a way to maintain a living in the absence of social security benefits and will improve the society's view of the aged. No longer will geriatric centers be greatly used as the aged now have valuable social status, and those facilities once reserved for the aged are now filled by the dying.
>
> Law and order in America may be severely stressed as a result of high medical costs and an absence of both health insurance or social welfare benefits for families left homeless and destitute from loss of the "bread winner." The resulting social stress placed on destitute survivors will doubtlessly increase crime rates. Police

> services will be overworked and undermanned. Families may be forced to become more directly responsible for their own protection. Vigilanteism may increase substantially with citizens not only protecting their possessions but also their health—AIDS victims may be persecuted by such groups. Social conditions will be "ripe" for the advent of extremist political groups searching for and, no doubt, finding a scapegoat group. Euthanasia within the AIDS victim community may become legally possible and encouraged in some areas.

Whether this, or an approximation of this, scenario develops is certainly contingent on a host of factors. The AIDS incidence rates in Africa where, within a few years, 50% of the population of some countries may die, might serve as a model for the future of the disease in the U.S. Certainly the level of sophistication of American health, education, and communications systems greatly surpasses that of the Third World nations and, thereby, suggests the AIDS epidemic may not decimate 50% of the American population. If health and education systems in America do not change American sexual behavior, regardless of America's sophistication, the writing may be on the wall. An appropriate question is: what is the social impact of AIDS in those African nations where it is now threatening a large percentage of the population?

The Geneva-based World Health Organization estimates that 2 million to 5 million Africans are now carriers of the AIDS virus. Leading researchers believe at least 50,000 people have already died of AIDS in Africa and unless a treatment and vaccine are found, a million and a half more may succumb over the next decade. That potential may face America and, if no vaccine/cure or change in societal sexual behavior occurs, may be only a weigh-station toward further slaughter.

The major transmission factor, promiscuity, combined with a higher incidence of venereal disease among Africans has apparently accelerated the spread of the AIDS virus—"some investigators have proposed that high rates of untreated venereal diseases in certain populations in Africa may enhance the efficiency of infection with HIV following exposure . . . such as syphilis, gonorrhea, or the presence of genital ulcers."[1] In some areas of Rwanda, Africa, which has a high incidence of AIDS, wives, as a method of birth control, avoid sex with their husbands for two years after a birth during which time husbands have sex with other women. This cultural method of birth control, effective in the past, is now decimating whole families. Forced urbanization and poverty in the region have also contributed to an increase in promiscuity as the population, in order to escape rural poverty and increase the chance of employment, has fled to densely populated cities where night life thrives and forms of prostitution and other illicit sex are commonplace.

Promiscuity as a Factor in AIDS Spread in America

According to Masters and Johnson, the incidence rate of gonorrhea in relation to promiscuity in the United States in 1980 approached only 460 in 100,000 with, however, much under-reporting. "More than a million [total] cases are reported annually [in the U.S.], and these probably represent only a quarter of the actual cases that occur each year." Because of under-reporting and the means of easy treatment for gonorrhea in the U.S., perhaps a better measure of potential AIDS impact on American society may exist in rates of genital herpes. "Genital herpes currently affects some 15 to 20 million Americans, with an additional 500,000 cases occurring annually."[2] Nearly half of the adult population in America now is infected by genital herpes—not an encouraging picture in relation to the potential spread of a sexually transmitted disease such as AIDS.

If the incidence rates of the sexually transmitted diseases in America are a valid predictor of AIDS's potential, the country may indeed lose between 30-50% of its adult population by 2010 with incalculable effect. In Africa, while nations have, so far, not been destabilized by AIDS, there are signs of trouble ahead. Most of the victims are young people between the ages of 19 and 40—the same age group as most commonly infected in the United States. At the very least, the potential for AIDS's impact on the young adult American population and its subsequent impact on the economy calls for national planning efforts to avert possible economic collapse. Planning efforts should be at least equal to that which are now being devoted to vaccine development.

The Need for Social Planning

To avoid planning or to assume that a "miracle bullet" will be developed which will avert a catastrophe such as the

United States has never seen, is to open the risk that American culture must regress to a level not seen since the late 1800s. The issues that national social planners must address appear truly awesome—virtually every social system in the nation will be effected. A national social planning strategy, however, requires first that a national policy toward the epidemic be drafted and as of 1987, the only broadly articulated national policy toward the disease states that everyone, particularly sexually active youngsters, should know that having sex without a condom (perhaps even with a condom) and/or spermicidal jelly is risking your life and that abstinence is the best policy. With bittersweet tongue in cheek abstinence does indeed appear to be the national policy—abstinence from traditional strategies of controlling a society-threatening invasion.

AIDS Dementia and Systems' Incompetencies

Another threat to the society, which shall surely intensify the necessity for action, is the fact that AIDS targets the brain cells of infected individuals directly causing progressive dementia. Even before numbers of deaths skyrocket (i.e., measured in millions), segments of society will see an escalating level of incompetency. It will appear primarily at first in currently highly infected population segments: the poor, under-educated minority groups, homosexuals, and intravenous drug abusers and eventually move into low-tech service and finally into the high-tech service industries. Essentially, escalating incompetency among groups should closely correlate to the educational level of those groups. How that escalating incompetency will be played out promises interesting social potentials. Progressive dementia among the undereducated segments of society may result in an increase in irrational criminal activity among those groups and, proportionately, larger cities of the nation may expect to see an escalation in property crimes and personal assaults—theft, robbery, and rape. The extent to which dementia among the under-educated will lead to an increase in crime will vary from city to city and be correlated both to the level of social services provided to this group and the level of law enforcement activities undertaken by a city.

Among low-tech service industries it is likely that municipal services, building trades, automotive services, food services, and transportation services may be among occupations next suffering from an escalating incompetency. Results of increased numbers of individuals suffering progressive dementia in these fields may translate into loss of efficiency in a city's infrastructure. It may not be unrealistic to expect problems in garbage collection, sewer and water maintenance, and perhaps in law enforcement. It appears prudent that cities may wish to require mandatory blood testing of municipal employees who have positions of responsibility which, if abused, could seriously affect large numbers of a city's population. Loss of competence among certain segments of the building trades could result in inferior and potentially dangerous buildings.

Automotive services' decline in effectiveness may result in unsafe vehicles. Declines in food services' effectiveness may contribute to the development of disease, e.g., salmonella. Transportation services' declines could result in selective shortages of goods. Finally, declines in effectiveness of high-tech services such as air traffic control, nuclear reactor operators, and chemical manufacturing employees could potentially result in extremely serious safety problems to large numbers of individuals.

Can we, in this interdependent and highly technological society, afford to allow employees in positions of high responsibility for/to large numbers of individuals practice their trades without some type of protection? What, for example, would be the legal resolution of a case where a city employee, suffering from dementia yet still capable of reporting to work, decides to poison the city in some misguided effort to revenge his/her own expected death? What would be the potential damage to life if the AIDS-demented operator of a nuclear power station decided to melt down the reactor? Certainly, with the potential of tens of millions eventually being infected by 1995, each passing year without development of a policy related to AIDS dementia and its relationship to high-responsibility employment increases the risk for needless accidents and subsequent legal liabilities.

AIDS and the Development of Extremist Groups

In any situation of national-level concern when the leadership of a country fails to provide effective solutions to a potentially catastrophic problem, history has shown that extremist groups profligate. One need only examine the Weimer Republic of Germany in the 1930s and the subsequent rise of the Nazis as evidence. Offering solutions to the economic woes of the nation as well as a convenient scapegoat, Hitler rose to power by the choice of the common citizen. In the 1790s, France, facing a hyperinflationary crisis, chose Napoleon as its leader. He then quickly put into action his megalomaniacal plans to conquer Europe. Both of these infamous leaders came to power by offering a radical solution, combined with effective oration, in a situation in which a nation was desperate for answers and where the existing governments had none.

The parallels to AIDS in the United States, though not yet immediately visible, are just around the corner. What if the national health care expenses for AIDS treatment approaches a $10 trillion total or even $600 billion annual cost? Where will the funding for this incredible expense come from? This capital must be developed in an environment where a huge percent of potential wage earners and subsequent tax payers will be either dead or incapacitated. As the national debt in 1987 is near $2 trillion and that debt has had the effect of increasing interest rates, what could be the effect on the economy with a $5-$10 trillion additional expense? Surely either a deflationary or hyperinflationary crisis will result with loss of purchasing power or ability of the general public and subsequent political unrest. Quite likely, the federal government may opt for hyperinflation knowing full well that it will eventually bankrupt the country but will allow repayment of debts with cheaper dollars in the short run. Imagine a 1987 $60,000 home costing $400,000 in 1997 with a variable interest rate at 35% and a 20% cap. Who could afford it? Who would be angry?

Potential for Revolution?

If the nation gets to this point, which all current trends appear to strongly suggest, civil disobedience will follow. If galvanized into a common will through the effective oration of radical solutions by a charismatic leader, America will be the France of the 1790s, the Germany of the 1930s. Revolution could be possible and who would be the scapegoat? Would it be the Jews as in the Black Death of the 1300s, or as it was in the 1940s?

Would it be the homosexual community, the Russians, immigrants, scientists, or big business? To be sure, if America goes through the future as it now appears to be going, there will be a scapegoat. Indications of the development of radical political elements will be more visible as a function of increasing deaths and subsequent effect on the economy. Vigilance is advised.

AIDS and Geopolitics

By the early 2000s the costs for AIDS care in America will be incredible, potentially equaling the total federal budget of 1985. (The nation will be forced into an economic corner of national defense—but will the true enemy be from without or from within.) To maintain a military budget comparable to that of 1987 (approximately $300 billion), while at the same time providing a social budget supportive of the AIDS-infected population (perhaps as much as $1 trillion per year by 2004) and continuing to pay interest on the national debt (perhaps $300-$500 billion per year by 2004) would require a tremendous increase in income taxes. Unfortunately, by 2004, the ranks of taxpaying citizens will have dwindled. The resultant economic environment may leave the federal government with the following possible choices:

	Military Spending	Social/Health Spending	National Debt Payments
1.	Y	Y	N
2.	Y	Y	Y
3.	Y	N	N
4.	Y	N	Y
5.	N	Y	N
6.	N	Y	Y
7.	N	N	N
8.	N	N	Y

(Y=yes; N=no)

With total costs and potentially available revenues essentially negating the possibility of option 2 above, reprioritization of expenditures seems apparent. To maintain military budgets either social/health budgets and/or payments of the national debt will be reduced or suspended. Ceasing payment on the national debt would result in a potential for hyperinflation and would increase inflation drastically. Reducing or limiting social/health budgets would result in a potential for emergence of political extremists. Finally, reducing military spending would result in a national security risk and reduced ability to project political power throughout the world. In short, there are limited choices ahead for the federal government and each choice is capable only of minimizing degradation of services. In no instance is there an apparent viable solution allowing a simultaneous beneficial solution. Geopolitical abilities of the United States may be reduced and stress to or instability of the government would be the result of any budgetary decision.

The federal government, being forced into a situation of extremely limited choice, may less cautiously begin to approach geopolitical issues. With half of the population already sentenced to eventual death by AIDS and with an inability to cope economically with that potential, why not risk war as a back door strategy to avoid facing responsibility? Particularly dangerous, this strategy may become more probable as a viable option if the government fails to reduce disease spread.

Epilogue

The potential impact of a runaway AIDS epidemic in America on the social fabric of the nation is frightening. Life in America may be like life in the late 1800s replete with the many societal changes therein associated. It is entirely possible that 30-50% of the adult population of the country may be felled by this disease. Its impact on the social fabric of the nation is incalculable.

As these changes occur and, depending upon the severity of national impact and mobilization, begin to cause a major decline in society, the level of generalized fear among the population may prove a fertile ground for any leader offering solutions. The impact of AIDS on the social fabric may create a political climate for installation of a totalitarian/authoritarian system of government. Also, the potential for hyperinflation or reduced geopolitical abilities and subsequent national security problems may be the result of an unchecked AIDS epidemic. The federal government must now develop strategies in anticipation of the probable economic impact resultant from the epidemic. The individual citizen must closely monitor the government's approach.

Notes

[1] Marlink, R. G., and Essex, M. "Africa and the Biology of Human Immunodeficiency Virus," *JAMA* 257.19: 2633.

[2] Masters, W.; Johnson, V. *Human Sexuality* (Boston, MA: Little Brown and Company,1985) 556.

AIDS: What Are Your Chances?

AIDS is numerically a very deceptive disease. Its current growth rate in most countries is "exponential" or "geometric." That type of growth is deceptive in that first reports of the disease are miniscule—provoking a common sentiment among the general population of "why worry about something so small." As time progresses the disease infects more people but still the risk to a given individual is small. However, there comes a point in time in an exponential increase when it seems the growth rate suddenly explodes.

Consider this analogy: You are paid $.01 per hour and each hour your pay doubles, e.g., your first hour you earn $.01; second hour $.02, third hour $.04 and so on. How much will you be paid per hour during the last hour of a 40 hour week? Answer: $5,497,558,139 per hour. This type of growth is what is now occurring in the AIDS epidemic. In terms of the above analogy, we the country, in 1987, are at the end of the first day of the week. The "week" ends in America by 2010 when, assuming AIDS continues its now evidenced growth, up to 180 million persons could be infected in this country alone.

An absurd possibility? The reports of concern discussed previously in this book suggest not. Even if the above projection is off by 75%, 45 million Americans may still be victims of the disease. We are, as Dr. Robert Gallo of the National Cancer Research Institut, has stated, on the edge of a great "plague."

> The word "plague" had just been uttered for the first time. At this stage of the narrative, with Dr. Benard Rieux standing at his window, the narrator may, perhaps, be allowed to justify the doctor's uncertainty and surprise—since with very slight differences, his reaction was the same as that of the great majority of our townsfolk. Everybody knows that pestilences have a way of recurring in the world; yet somehow we find it hard to believe in ones that crash down on our heads from a blue sky. There have been as many plagues as wars in history; yet plagues and wars always take people equally by surprise.
>
> In fact, like our fellow citizens, Rieux was caught off his guard and we should understand his hesitations in the light of this fact;

> and similarly understand how he was torn between conflicting fears and confidence. When a war breaks out, people say: "It's too stupid; it can't last long." But though a war may well be "too stupid," that doesn't prevent its lasting. Stupidity has a knack of getting its way; as we should see if we were not always so much wrapped up in ourselves.
>
> In this respect, out townsfolk were like everybody else wrapped up in themselves; in other words they were humanists: they disbelieved in pestilences. A pestilence isn't a thing made to man's measure; therefore we tell ourselves that pestilence is a mere bogy of the mind, a bad dream that will pass away. But it doesn't always pass away and from one bad dream to another it is men who pass away, and the humanists first of all, because they haven't taken their precautions. Our townsfolk were not more to blame than others; they forgot to be modest, that was all and thought that everything still was possible for them; which presupposed that pestilences were impossible. They went on doing business, arranged for journeys, and formed views. How should they have given a thought to anything like plague, which rules out any future, cancels journeys, silences the exchange of views. They fancied themselves free, and no one will ever be free so long as there are pestilences.
>
> From *The Plague*, by Albert Camus

Death by AIDS

You have probably not seen a person dying of AIDS and have no conception of the type of death AIDS brings. You have probably not yet made any significant changes in your sexual behavior if those changes are necessary. You may not have given much thought to the potentials of AIDS at all and you may even be avoiding thinking about it. If you are not now infected and if you are saying "This won't happen to me" and if you are engaging in sexual activity with more than one other person who you know is not infected, then within the next few years this may be you:

> You are lying in a hospital bed suffering from pneumonia for the 3rd time. People you know do not come to visit you and you can sense among the staff caring for you that they are uneasy. Your body is covered with purple raised patches of Kaposi's sarcoma—a skin cancer. You cannot easily breathe and at times you become frightened that you may suffocate. Your memory and concentration powers are waning—the result of the virus's assault on your brain tissue. You are easily nauseated, vomiting has become standard. You have constant diarrhea. You cough and sneeze. You have had

> times when you have urinated and defecated in your bed and when someone came to assist you they were dressed up with gowns, caps, gloves and goggles as if you were radioactive. Every tissue you use must be placed in a special container. You think, "why me?" You must ponder your own death. To move becomes incredibly painful; your skin is cracked and sore. You may think about suicide. Disease after disease racks your body. The illness is so weird. You've never heard of it before. You're angry and depressed: what will happen to your family; your children, why?

It takes between 18 months to 3 years to die from AIDS after you have been diagnosed but, so far it is certain you will die. No one has survived AIDS.

Avoiding AIDS

To avoid contracting this disease you must simply take responsibility for your own behavior. There are specific activities which you must not do in order to reduce your risk. What are they? Specifically you must:

1. Avoid sexual contact with a number of persons—keep numbers to a minimum.

2. Avoid anal copulation.

3. Avoid vaginal intercourse with anyone who has possibly had sexual contact with others.

4. Avoid fellatio or cunnilingus with anyone who has possibly had sexual contact with others.

5. Avoid french kissing with anyone who has possibly had sexual contact with others.

6. Avoid contact with any body fluid from anyone you do not know, who has not been recently tested for AIDS, or who might have had sexual contact with others.

7. Maintain a *strictly* monogamous relationship.

8. If you desire to have sexual contact with a new partner, insist

that this partner take a blood test for the virus.

9. Avoid sexual contact with a new person who has blood tested *negative* for AIDS for at least 3 months and then insist that that person retest negative again. During that 3 month period that person must not have had sexual contact with any person.

10. In those cases where you insist on sexual contact, use a condom, a diaphragm and monoxynol-9 (a spermicide) carefully, but *be aware* that this protection may fail and you may contract AIDS.

11. Avoid sharing needles or syringes with anyone if you use IV drugs.

12. Avoid sexual contact with persons who use IV drugs.

13. Avoid sexual contact with prostitutes.

14. Avoid sharing razor blades, toothbrushes, or other implements that could become contaminated with blood.

15. Avoid sexual contact with persons known or suspected of having AIDS.

16. Avoid oral, vaginal, or anal contact with semen.

17. Avoid contact with a partner's urine in mouth, anus, eyes, or open cuts or sores.

18. Avoid insertion of fingers or fists into the anus as active or receptive partner.

19. Avoid oral contact with the anus.

Your own personal risk of contracting AIDS is, to a great extent, a direct result of your own behavior. To avoid thinking about the risk of AIDS with any and every sexual contact—that which is not a long-established monogamous relationship—is equivalent to playing Russian roulette. The only difference is that with Russian roulette you die instantly and not over a 2-3 year period of progressive suffering.

As the number of AIDS cases and unidentified infected

persons escalates—as both will—the absolute necessity of your control of your sexual behavior will escalate. By 1991 it has been estimated that 10 million Americans will be infected by the virus—by 2001 perhaps 50 million. It cannot be emphasized enough that you will *probably die from AIDS within 20 years if you do not now change your sexual behavior.*

Increased Concerns About the Blood Supply

"America's blood supply, already being screened for the AIDS virus might be facing a threat from another potentially deadly virus—HTLV-I. The American Red Cross is sampling blood donated by more than 30,000 people in the Los Angeles metropolitan area and five unidentified cities to see if a rare virus capable of causing a particularly deadly form of leukemia and possibly a nerve disease is being spread through transfusions."[1] The HTLV-I virus according to Dr. Bernard Poiesz, a State University of New York medical professor, has invaded the blood supply. He stated, "The number of Americans infected . . . is already in the thousands, possibly tens of thousands [and resembles AIDS because it] causes an almost universally fatal disease."[2] It is transmitted by blood transfusions, sharing infected needles and during sexual intercourse. The HTLV-I leukemia appears to take an average of four years to manifest its symptoms, but once seen, kills its victims quickly—usually within three months.

An Increase in Other Communicable Diseases

Substantial evidence has developed showing that some AIDS victims are developing tuberculosis which *can* be transmitted through casual contact. In the very near future more information about this may be presented to the general public further raising concern. There may be an increase in intestinal diseases due to an environment conducive to proliferating viral infections of all types.

Finally, another AIDS relative, LAV-2/HIV-2 (lymphoadenopathy-associated virus type 2) has been recently reported by Luc Montagnier, of the Pasteur Institute in Paris, and has been found to cause AIDS in some West African patients.[3] Montagneir stated, "Clearly, this virus (HIV-2) is also pathogenic in man . . . it could be just a matter of time [before this new AIDS virus also becomes epidemic]."[4] Montagneir may be right as the HIV-2 virus has begun to spread outside of West Africa.

Epilogue

That you are responsible through your own sexual behavior for your health and the future of this nation cannot be overemphasized. As the only means to avert a national tragedy of a type the nation has never known, your own education and responsible action in the AIDS pandemic can be considered a patriotic act. The AIDS epidemic is no joke. Even if you yourself do not contract the virus, you will be greatly affected by the societal changes that will surely occur unless or until people collectively change their sexual behavior.

Further affecting your chances, another retrovirus (HTLV-I) appears to have made its way into the nation's blood supply along with HTLV-III/LAV. In conjunction with your responsible sexuality, another method of reducing your risk for AIDS and other blood-borne viruses appears to be the pre-donation of your own blood for your own use in the event it is required by you.

Your responsible action is to educate those persons with whom you have contact and to control your own sexual behavior. If you act, then you can avoid a prolonged suffering death. If the nation acts then we can avoid a potential prolonged suffering collapse into totalitarianism or anarchy.

Notes

1 Greenwalt, F. "Newest Threat to Blood Supply," *Daily News* [Los Angeles, California] Jan. 21, 1987.

2 Nicholson, J. "Deadly New Cancer 'Spreading like AIDS,'" *New York Post* Jan. 21, 1987.

[3] Barnes, D. M. "Broad Issues Debated at AIDS Vaccine Workshop," *Science* 236.4799: 256.

[4] Edwards, D. D. "AIDS Researchers Debate Danger of HIV-2," *Science News* March 7, 1987: 151.

AIDS: Progress Toward Vaccines/Treatment

AIDS is proving to be a difficult vaccine-development problem. The genetic structure of HTLV-III/LAV varies considerably from one strain to another, and an effective vaccine would have to protect against all the strains. Some researchers believe that AIDS may be caused by a family of closely related viruses, further complicating vaccine development. Even so, French researchers in Zaire are already testing a prototype vaccine. Whether that trial vaccine is effective will hopefully be known in 1988.

To further discourage the possibility of a quick victory, AIDS vaccine development may be compared to development of a cancer vaccine. "The fight against AIDS is looking more and more like cancer pharmacology, a long, tedious, and expensive process"[1] making the rapid discovery of a vaccine unlikely. Additionally, the experimental testing necessities of vaccine development such as ethics, use and location of human subjects, and federal regulation problems will likely delay speedy development of a vaccine.

Because the AIDS virus is not just one virus but a continually mutating series of closely related viruses, development of a vaccine is much like shooting in the dark at a moving target. Surgeon General Koop has stated that it may not be until the turn of the century before a safe and effective vaccine for AIDS is available for the general population. Dr. Robert Gallo has remarked, "The way we see the virus now is that there aren't strains—A, B and C—but rather a continuum of virus isolates."[2] Some researchers believe that an effective vaccine for AIDS may *never* be possible.

To further confound quick development of a vaccine, the virus itself, because of the extremely slow development of symptoms in a victim, makes determination of the effectiveness of any vaccine impossible for perhaps 5 years *after the vaccine has been administered* and that much time must pass before an individual may show symptoms of the disease. With the legal precedential issues concerning drug companies being sued for product failure, the time when a vaccine can be delivered to the general public may be lengthened. According to Surgeon General Koop it may be at least 18 years before an effective vaccine is available. Additionally, with HTLV-I, tuberculosis, intestinal viruses, LAV-2 and now HIV-3 (another AIDS-causing retrovirus reported found in Nigeria, Africa) becoming potential threats as well, research budgets for vaccine development may be widely diffused.

At a recent (March 25-27, 1987) scientific workshop on AIDS vaccines sponsored by the U. S. Department of Public Health, many questions arose regarding the logistics of AIDS vaccine development. Among the questions arising at this workshop were: 1. Should vaccines be developed which prevent infection of a non-infected person?; should a vaccine be used to prevent the deterioration of an infected person's health to the point where full-blown AIDS develops?; and should vaccines be given to persons who now have AIDS? 2. Who should be given a candidate AIDS vaccine?; how should clinical trials for testing a candidate vaccine be constructed?; and what of product liability and the ethics of administering candidate vaccines?; 3. How will it be known that the candidate vaccine is effective?; should candidate vaccines be tested on chimpanzees or other species?, will results of vaccine effectiveness be applicable to human subjects?

Quite literally, the questions that are being asked by these pre-eminent AIDS researchers are the most basic questions in the long process of vaccine development. As of March 1987, some researchers continue to doubt that a vaccine will ever exist for AIDS due to the speed at which the AIDS retrovirus mutates.[3]

According to the Food and Drug Administration, during late March 1987, three U. S. research groups applied for permission to begin human testing of their respective candidate vaccines despite the fact that *no* studies of candidate vaccines have been found to protect chimpanzees (the only other laboratory test animal besides the rhesus macque known to be able to be infected by the AIDS virus). Many scientists have expressed concern that testing of candidate vaccines should demonstrate protection from the virus in chimpanzees before human tests begin. A poignant comment made at the AIDS vaccine workshop emphasizes caution, "Once we start down the road of giving vaccines to humans, how far can we go without knowing that they (candidate vaccines) are efficacious? The public pressure to push on will be considerable."[4]

In short, the quick development of a vaccine, such as was seen during the 1950's for polio, is not likely to occur. Barring a scien-tific breakthrough, the process of developing an effective vaccine will, at best, be long and, at worst, will fail. AIDS is caused by the HTLV-III/LAV/HIV retrovirus families and according to Dr. Anthony Fauci, director of the National Institute of Allergy and Infectious Diseases, "We know very little about man's protection against a retrovirus."[5] No vaccine for any human retrovirus has ever been developed and, according to Dr. Dani Bolognesi, of Duke University, "We're at the beginning of this. We're at stage one and it's a multistep process."[6] Dr. Martin Malcomb, of the National Institute of Allergy and Infectious Diseases stated, "The more we know [about the HTLV-III/LAV retrovirus] the less we know."[7]

Development of a Cure?

Complicating potential cure development is evidence that the HTLV-III/LAV virus not only spreads from person to person but to different cell types within a person. The virus may remain hidden within those other cell types being protected by the cells' membranes from potential curing antibody attack. Hypothetically, the AIDS virus could "hideout" in cells until antibody levels from any "cure" decline and then, once again, become active. Such viral action may require continual booster antibody injections to keep the disease in check.

In almost a full circle, Dr. Robert C. Gallo, co-discoverer of the HTLV-III/LAV retrovirus, predicted on March 25, 1987 that no cure for AIDS would be found in our lifetime. In a poll of 227 scientists conducted by Louis Harris & Associates for the Bristol Myers pharmaceutical firm, 52 percent of reporting scientists said they expected a cure for AIDS by the year 2010. At best, it appears a cure may not be available until the disease has decimated the population.

Even though knowledge about the virus has advanced tremendously since its isolation in 1983, there are indications that some of the relatively more simple mechanisms of HTLV-III/LAV are not yet understood. Richard Axel, of the College of Physicians and Surgeons of Columbia University, and Robin Weiss, of the Chester Beatty Laboratories in London, have suggested that there may still be molecules used by the virus to bind to cells not yet discovered. What is known for certain is that cells attacked by HTLV-III/LAV have the antigen CD4 present on their surfaces to which the virus can bind, but certain brain cells attacked by HIV do not have the CD4 antigen on their surface, suggesting the virus may be able to bind to cells which possess some other as yet unidentified receptor or antigen. Dr. John Ziegler and Dr. Daniel P. Stites of the University of California at San Francisco have suggested that perhaps a vaccine which would effectively kill the AIDS virus could also kill noninfected immunogenic cells which "lock" with CD4 cells and help trigger an immune response—essentially a vaccine could trigger an immune deficiency in an individual by killing off necessary cells which the AIDS virus appears to mimic. Much is known about HIV, but many mysteries remain.

Treatment for AIDS

Drugs potentially helpful in treating AIDS may include ribavirin, azidothymidine, HPA 23, foscarnet, TP-1, interferon, and interleukin. Other drugs include phosphonoformate, BW A5094, Compound S, dideoxycytidine, ansamycin, isoprinosine, thymopectin, gamma interferon, interleukin-2 as well as AL721, ampligen, ansamycin, azimexon, cyclosporine, imreg-1, inosine pranobex, and d-penicillamine. The degree of effectiveness and toxicity of these drugs is often not well known and prescribing them for a treatment may be hazardous.

AZT as a Treatment of AIDS

AZT (3'-azido-3'-deoxythymidine) is not a cure for AIDS, although study results hold great promise for prolonging life for certain patients with AIDS. Uncertainties about AZT remain: uncertainties about possible toxic effects and uncertainties about long-term benefits or ill effects. "The potential effectiveness of AZT, as well as its potential toxicity, are simply unknown over the long term. It remains, however, the only therapy for AIDS that has shown even partial effectiveness."[8]

So far, the most serious toxic effect of AZT is inhibition of the normal production of red blood cells by the bone marow.

Forty patients who received AZT (in clinical trials) required transfusions for anemia, compared to 11 patients from a placebo group needing transfusions, suggesting AZT may deplete the red blood cells in patients. Another common side effect of AZT is headaches. "In addition to decreasing the mortality rate of AIDS patients with *pneumocystis* pneumonia, at least over the short term, AZT also seems to improve their quality of life. To varying degrees, AZT recipients had fewer serious medical complications, showed an increase in the number of circulating T4-leukocytes, could respond to a mild immune stimulus in a skin test, and had an improved sense of well-being.[9] However, Michael Osterholm, Minnesota state epidemiologist, reported in the *St. Paul Pioneer Press-Dispatch,* "Its [AZT's] effects are, at best, short-lived . . . It isn't the answer. It's a first step. It would be unfortunate if people thought this was the panacea."[10] It appears that in half of the cases where AZT is given to an AIDS patient the drug must be stopped because of its toxicity.

AZT blocks the ability of the AIDS virus to replicate inside a host cell. It interrupts elongation of chains of DNA, making it impossible for the virus to complete DNA synthesis and thus reproduce itself. But how these molecular events, which were initially deduced by studying the action of AZT on virus-infected cells growing in laboratory culture dishes, translate into the clinical improvement of AIDS patients is still not clear. Now available for the general population of AIDS victims from Burroughs-Wellcome Laboratories, the costs for AZT may be prohibitive and quantities may be difficult to obtain.

Other Potential Treatments

DDC, developed by Hoffmann-LaRoche, is a sister drug to AZT and appears extremely promising in laboratory experiments. Although DDC has only been tested on a small population, the drug may prove to be more potent and less toxic than AZT.

AL721, a drug developed by Praxis Pharmaceuticals to ease the symptoms of drug withdrawal, is in very early trials to determine its effectiveness against AIDS. With a very small sample population, the AL721 seems to have reduced swelling of the lymph nodes in some AIDS patients. AL721 appears to interfere with the infectiousness of the AIDS virus, possibly by attacking the virus' outer envelope. No side effects were found during a six-week trial in humans.

Granulocyte-monocyte colony-stimulating factor (GCF), by Genetics Institute, has shown promise in treating AIDS in animals. Any results from human-based research of GCF will not be available until late 1987.

Alpha interferon, from several pharmaceutical companies (Biogen; Schering-Plough; Hoffmann-LaRoche; and Genen-tech), has shown promise as an effective treatment of Kaposi's sarcoma.

Research at present is focusing on the effectiveness of alpha interferon in combination with AZT. Interleukin-2, by Hoffmann-LaRoche and Immunex Cetus, has generally been disappointing when IL-2 is used by itself as a treatment. Researchers are, however, beginning to test Interleukin-2 in combination with AZT as a treatment. No human test results are currently available. Cyclosporine, by Sandoz, is a highly toxic drug that is used to prevent a person's immune system from rejecting transplanted tissue. Some French researchers have discovered that, in the early stages of AIDS, cyclosporine seems to control the growth of the AIDS virus in patients. Its method of help is centered on a suppression of the immune system and subsequent lack of stimulation of AIDS-infected T4-cells which, thereby, prohibits growth of more AIDS virions.

What Triggers the Onset of Full-Blown AIDS?

Research is being done in those individuals who are infected by the virus but not yet showing major symptoms. Research is being conducted to determine what triggers the onset of full-blown AIDS. Theories are varied. Some researchers suggest subsequent viral infection (any of a multitude) of HTLV-III/LAV seropositive individuals will provoke onset of the disease. Still others suggest that there may be a genetic predisposition in some individuals for eventually developing the disease—particularly in individuals whose "keyed" immune system cells (normally "locking" up with CD4 cells and triggering activation of the immune system) genetically closely resemble the AIDS virus. The theory continues that the antibodies produced naturally by the body to attack the AIDS virus then also attack these "keyed" cells and eventually CD4 cells directly, resulting in the self-destruction of the immune system—a kind of Lupus Disease of the Immune system. If true, this theory suggests that a genetic marker could be found which could discover those HTLV-III/LAV seropositive individuals who would go on to develop full-blown AIDS.

Bureaucratic Problems in Development of Treatment

Finally, some critics of the federal effort in the development of treatment cite bureaucratic inefficiency as a major hinrance to the development of effective treatment for AIDS. Mathilde Krim, co-chair of the American Foundation for AIDS Re-search in New York City, stated in January 1987, "There is very little going on [regarding treatment developments] and what they [the National Institute for Allergy and Infectious Diseases (NIAID) in Bethesda, MD.] are doing is peanuts. The whole thing (organization) is a mess."[11] And Jeffrey Levi, executive director of the National Gay and Lesbian Task Force in Washington, D. C., also critical of NIAID, complained that they are slow to start, which he regarded as inexcusable.

Dr. Arnold Lippa, president of Praxis Pharmaceuticals of Los Angeles (the firm working on development of AL721) said "We have waited three months since we submitted the data for them to say something [regarding starting clinical trials of AL721] and we can no longer anticipate any assistance from the federal government and are planning large clinical trials on our own."[12] Simply, in regard to development of possible treatments, the federal government has seemingly slowed efforts through inefficient organization.

"Snake Oil" Treatments and AIDS

Every time there is a serious disease—especially one that's as lethal as AIDS—the darker side of human nature is revealed. Inevitably, there will be some people willing to prey on those who have the disease or who are afraid of getting it. In this epidemic, salesmen of "miracle medicine" have already begun bilking dying patients of their remaining funds.

A Dallas-based nutrition firm, United Sciences of America, Inc., now under Chapter 11 bankruptcy, sold "an estimated $27 million worth of products it claimed could prevent AIDS and treat or prevent a variety of other illnesses." Two different products sold by this firm, "Fiber Energy Bar" and "Master Formula" were purported by United Sciences to "prevent AIDS, delay deterioration of the immune system, lower cholesterol, help diabetics and lower the incidence of heart disease"[13] as well as a host of other claims.

Other bogus products have been reported by the FDA to have seen sold for AIDS's treatment or prevention including a substance called "R'Bella" in Washington, D. C., which was determined to be a traditional douche relabeled as a miracle drug; "ZPG-1," an "anti-aids" pill made from zinc glutamate and sold in New York; and a rather bizarre treatment, provided by William Hitt, in Texas, of injecting AIDS patients with their own "ultra-filtered" urine.

As the numbers of infected grow it is reasonable to expect that more "miracle drugs" sold by the unethical will increase and that a black market for "cures" will develop. Many infected persons, desperate for help, will be gouged of their remaining life's savings. Caution is advised.

Epilogue

The search for an effective vaccine is under progress and is a research priority among many molecular biologists. Barring a scientific breakthrough it is unlikely that an effective vaccine will be available before the "turn of the century" according to Surgeon General C. Everett Koop. Further, if a vaccine were shown to be effective in clinical trials today, it would likely be 5-7 years before it would reach the public. Research on a prototype vaccine is being tested by the French in Zaire, Africa, but results of those tests will not be known for some time.

As of March 1987, the only drug available for treatment of AIDS is AZT which is only effective with some patients. The drug has some documented toxic effects in other patients, requiring relatively frequent blood transfusions. The drug is costly, hard to obtain and must be taken every 4 hours for the rest of an AIDS victim's life. Other treatments are under investigation but it may be some time before any of these reach the general public. Many worthless "cures" will likely be seen in the black market.

The search for a vaccine/treatment of AIDS is proving to be a very difficult, costly and time-consuming scientific venture. Although the progress made thus far in understanding the virus has been without precedent in the annals of medicine, the HTLV-III/LAV/HIV virus will not give up its secrets easily, and development of an effective vaccine would be a scientific first for the human retroviruses. Probably a truly effective cure for AIDS will not be forthcoming for perhaps decades. Any cure may require use of retroviral in-vivo genetic engineering—a technology not yet possessed by the medical research community.

Notes

1 Nulty, P. "Drug Companies Fight the Dragon," *Fortune* Sept. 15, 1986: 133.

2 Dusheck, J. "HTLV-III virus: Themes and Variations," *Science News* 128.8: 119.

3 Barnes, D. M. "Broad Issues Debated at AIDS Vaccine Workshop," *Science* 236.4799:. 255.

4 Weisburd, S. "AIDS Vaccine: Time for Human Tests?, *Science News* April 4, 1987: 213.

5 Barnes, D. M. "Strategies for an AIDS Vaccine," *Science* 233.4769: 1153.

6 Barnes, "Strategies" 1149.

7 Silberner, J. "What Triggers AIDS?," *Science News* April 4, 1987: 220.

8 Barnes, D. M. "Promising Results Halt Trial of Anti-AIDS Drug," *Science* 234.4772: 15.

9 Barnes 15-16.

10 Monsour, T. "Less Effective Than First Thought," *St. Paul (Minnesota) Pioneer Press-Dispatch*, Jan. 11, 1987.

11 Steinbrook, R. "Federal AIDS Effort Lages, Called a 'Mess' by Critics," *Los Angeles (California) Times*, Jan. 30, 1987.

12 Steinbrook, R.

13 Price, J. "Public Besieged by 'Drugs' That Don't Work." *Washington D.C. Times* Feb. 24, 1987.

AIDS: Where Do We Go From Here?

This is not a time for denying the potential realities of the AIDS epidemic—neither is it a time to panic about these potential realities. Our appropriate response should be control of our own sexual behavior and education of those persons around us. We must force our government to confront this problem now with logical planning and appropriately interventive public health, welfare and education strategies. With luck, changed sexual behavior, and an appropriate governmental response to the AIDS epidemic, deaths in the U. S. can be "minimized" (i.e., 2-5 million deaths). To continue the present course will result in the deaths of many more U. S. citizens and the devastation of our cities.

"Where do we go from here?" is a question not easily answered. The potential ramifications of a full-blown AIDS epidemic in this country are incalculable. Questions that must be addressed and areas that will certainly be effected vary from the individual to the world. What effect will a full-blown AIDS epidemic, resulting in millions of U. S. deaths, have on the American economy, the national debt, deficit, and value of the currency? What effect will an AIDS epidemic have on social welfare, social security, national health insurance, and the homeless? What effect will an AIDS epidemic have on the American family, the nation's educational systems, its criminal justice system, and law? What effect will an AIDS epidemic have on business, employment, transportation, and the production of goods and services? What effect will an AIDS epidemic have on our constitutional freedoms? These areas must be addressed.

Even more urgent, what effect will an AIDS epidemic have on national security, geopolitical stability, and rational leadership? Certainly, because of the impending number of worldwide casualties from this disease, any logical government would NOW be spending unprecedented sums to anticipate the near-term future, planning contingencies for coping with events, and providing massive public education such as has not been witnessed in modern society.

Is AIDS a Discriminatory Disease?

Barara Amiel, writing in *Maclean's* states, "Had the disease (AIDS) first been associated with white heterosexuals instead of Africans, Haitians and homosexuals, it is certainly my view that our policies toward this lethal epidemic would have been swift and unequivocal. The disease would have been notifiable to health authorities in all provinces in order to accurately monitor its spread. That notification would have included seropositive results, which could then be closely watched to determine what percentage of carriers develop full blown AIDS. AIDS cases would have been quarantined and there would have been no hesitation in protecting schoolchildren from infected playmates."[1] Perhaps she is right, and if she is, this epidemic, allowed to develop through latent racist and sexist attitudes, will repay that discrimination with a vengence.

Consider AIDS distribution by race and sex in Houston, Texas: 9.5% are black and 8.8% are Hispanic. 68% of blacks with AIDS are heterosexual and 22% of Hispanics with AIDS are heterosexual. Black women are 13-15 time more likely to have AIDS than white women.[2] Nationally the distribution for AIDS: in males is 63% white, 22% black and 14% Hispanic; in females is 27% white, 52% black, and 20% Hispanic. Is lack of effective intervention the result of viewing the epidemic as a problem of minorities?

A Most Frightening Type of Discrimination?

Perhaps the most frightening type of potential discrimination resulting from the AIDS epidemic is that which will surely occur if no substantial slowing of the disease occurs. Evidence has been presented that some of the most likely decimated groups of our society will be those which are now arguing for preservation of their civil rights. In essence, an argument can be made that current civil rights efforts are, in some respects preserving an ultimate civil right—the right to choose to die.

Certainly the free choice of those groups, i. e., to preserve the longer term option of death, must be protected. That choice, however, must not be one which is forced wholesale on other groups which have no vocal representation, e.g.., drug abusers and children. The long-term preservation of civil rights of any group may, in fact, be achieved through powerfully decisive intervention strategies. To argue against strong intervention based on scientific and logical methods seems both shortsighted and essentially egotistic—a result of the "me" generation of the 1970s.

What is Ethical in The Short and Long Term?

William F. Buckley Jr., editor of the *National Review* and host of the television program *Firing Line*, in a discussion with Dr. Alan Dershowitz suggested persons testing seropositive for AIDS be "tattooed discreetly, to guard uncontaminated sexual or needle partners from danger."[3] His comment was quickly branded as a Nazi-like suggestion and one which he has since recanted. But in the longer term this strategy, if carried out appropriately, may with sufficient confidentiality and legal controls, protect civil liberties of all groups of individuals. It would surely be at variance with traditional American views of privacy but such a method could preserve the ultimate freedom—that of choosing to live or die.

As of 1987, the American population is not sufficiently aware of the potential destructiveness of AIDS to our society. Any effort to either propose or implement strategically powerful interventions to curtail spread of the disease will provoke resistance. When enough of the general population become infected with AIDS, perhaps as little as 5% or 11 million persons, there will be a call from society at large to implement whatever methods are necessary to stop the spread of the disease. At current growth rates, that critical number of infected individuals will arrive sometime near 1994—just 7 years from now. Conceivably, the next U. S. President may be in a situation where greatly restrictive executive national security orders will be necessary.

The choices being made now, with the majority of Americans not having a sufficient understanding of the disease's impact, will dictate potential choices in the future. AIDS will not simply go away. We cannot just ignore it and expect that it will disappear. We cannot "turn the channel" to something more pleasant. And most assuredly, we cannot do just nothing. A choice to do nothing, whether by design or default, is in fact a choice. As has been amply presented in this book, our present course, and the decisions now dictating that course, is based on denial—our current choice is not to make a choice and as a result the scenarios outlined herein are quite likely to become reality. If by 1994, a call to action is finally demanded by society, many of the choices that "could have been" will be just that. Our options as a nation will be increasingly limited and the outcomes of interventions will be increasingly mutually exclusive requiring exceedingly more difficult choices.

We have said that the nation and the world are in a race against time. Perhaps a better analogy is that we are much like an ant trapped in the concave pit of the antlion. As of 1987 we have been slowly yet inexorably falling toward the awaiting jaws of the predator and with each month that passes without substantial intervention more sand falls down upon us and we are pushed closer to the bottom. Our options for escape become more limited.

An Avoidance-Avoidance Conflict

The nation is in an "avoidance" conflict. We wish to avoid assaults on civil rights but we also wish to avoid the economic and social disaster that may come. Typically, the result of an avoidance-avoidance conflict, whether individual or national, is to do nothing substantial to resolve the conflict—precisely what is happening now. The only way for that type of conflict to be resolved is to eventually choose that which is the least aversive of the options—and *not* choosing provokes anxiety. We are currently entering that time of intensified anxiety as we see no substantial reduction in the growth of the disease and we will continue to become even more anxious until the anxiety of non-choice is worse than either of the two alternatives.

Flawed Strategies?

Currently, strategies for trying to awaken the general public without provoking a panic are, when examined in light of avoidance-avoidance conflicts, doomed to failure. Sufficient anxiety will provoke action and very likely that action will be to choose reduction of civil rights rather than the destruction of

American social systems. An argument can be supported that a shorter term defense of individual civil rights threatens collective civil rights in the longer term.

The major problem with the strategy of raising concern yet preventing panic is that it is wasting valuable time and allowing the disease to make major inroads into the general population. Further, the strategy insures that polarization will develop in American society regarding what is the "worse of the two evils" i. e., preservation of society's rights at the expense of the individual's or preservation of the individual's rights at the expense of society's rights. Polarization of society is exactly what we, as a nation do not need as we face this, the most serious epidemic in the history of the world. As has been previously stated, that polarization, creating a volatile public, will provide an environment ripe for the advent of a totalitarian/ authoritarian form of government. This scenario is not without historic precedent. People will pay attention to anyone who has a "guaranteed" plan for stopping the disease.

In very clear terms, where we go from here can be simplified as follows: we can act decisively now and suffer a minimum of social and economic disruption yet maintain a system of government fairly similar to that which now exists, or we can refuse to act decisively now and suffer a maximum of social and economic disruption and lose that system of government with which we are familiar. The outcome of where we go from here is based in the final analysis on the interpretation of what AIDS can do to this country. Will it be a modern plague and kill half or more of our nation's population and reduce American social systems to memories of what was, or is AIDS and its potential impact just another false alarm sounded by doomsayers? Time will tell.

Epilogue

We as a society must be aware of the dire potentials of this disease. That awareness must not only include the need for individual prescriptive behavior changes, but the potential impact of AIDS on all systems of the American society. Current public policy must be intelligently weighed on the scale of long term potentials. Without education, people young and old in our country will likely continue to engage in high-risk sexual behavior and the government will not be motivated by grassroot political pressure to mount an aggressive unprecedented assault on the disease. With AIDS, what we don't know can not only kill us but kill our nation.

Notes

[1] Amiel, B. "The Politics of a Killer Disease," *Maclean's* Dec. 8, 1986: 11.

[2] Linthicum, L. "Minorities Learning of Danger From AIDS," *Houston (Texas) Post*, Jan. 5, 1987.

[3] Buckley, W. F. "The AIDS Battle Needs More Than Alarm Ringing," *Moline (Illinois) Daily Dispatch*, April 23, 1987: 4.

AIDS: Is There a Moral?

This unprecedented plague, resulting in many unknowns and consequent growing fear, is and will continue to become subject to moralistic interpretations. Those interpretations will be as wide ranging as will be the proposed alternatives for attacking the disease—each interpretation will serve as a philosophical underpinning of a proposed action. Simply, in a distilled view of potential moralistic interpretations/philosophies of the AIDS epidemic, there appears possible the following matrix of underpinning philosophies—each of which will determine the "world view" and actions of societal segments:

	Natural Cause	Divine Cause	Human Cause
By Design	Y	N	N
	N	Y	N
	N	N	Y
	N	N	N
By Accident	Y	N	N
	N	-	N
	N	N	Y
	N	N	N

(Y=yes; N=no)

Natural Cause by Design

The "Gaia Hypothesis," a theory held by some scientists, makes the assumption that the Earth is a living being with self-regulatory capabilities. The theory argues that, in the event of a continued insult to the Earth, self-regulatory processes will be set into action which attempt to purge the Earth of those continued insults. Such insults capable of provoking self-regulatory processes are to be found in repeated ecological assaults as well as high levels of negative, destructive thinking produced by a population dwelling in the afflicted areas. The interested reader is advised to research the Gaia Hypothesis.

Resultant moralizing based on a Gaia Hypothesis assumption will argue that AIDS is a result of the Earth's attempt to purge itself of the insults wrought by environmental assaults and the absence of positive, beneficial thought in societies. A prescriptive intervention based on this assumption for dealing with the AIDS epidemic may include the institution of strict environmental protections and strict codes of behavior designed to improve the collective society's thought patterns. The view may urge individual responsibility and focus on both behavioral and cognitive change.

Divine Cause by Design

"To travel around this country talking to people about AIDS is to learn quickly that many Americans still regard the emergence of the disease, which struck gays first, as an act of God. Even many comparatively free thinkers take the attitude that liberal Democrats did as they watched the cast of Watergate characters come to trial: 'I could have *told* you this was going to happen."[1] Whether AIDS is, in fact, some type of Divine judgment bears logical consideration in the sense that the epidemic is the direct result of the nation's collective non-responsible sexual behavior.

In examination of U. S. demographics of areas that have, from a religious standpoint, been traditionally considered "immoral" some support of a Divine judgment may exist—again, in the sense of that the disease is a result of non-responsible sexuality. Consider the following:

1. In 1982 19.4% of all births in the United States were to unmarried women, with the major contributors to that figure consisting of women between the ages of 15-24 years. The percent in 1950 was 3.9%.

2. In 1984 the ratio of divorce to marriages was 46.66%. In 1950 that ratio was 23.42%.

3. In 1982 .27% of all live births were from mothers less than 15 years of age In 1950 .15% of all live births were from mothers less than 15 years of age.

4. In 1981, the ratio of the number of abortions to the number of women aged 15-44 years old was 2.93%. In 1972, the ratio was 1.32%.

While these statistics, in themselves, say nothing conclusively, it appears that in all categories the reported behaviors appear to have nearly doubled from the '50s to the '80s.

In the *King James Bible,* the book of Deuteronomy, chapter 28, verses 58-62 provide a warning which could be construed by some to apply to the AIDS epidemic in America:

> "If thou wilt not observe to do all the words of this law that are written in this book, that thou mayest fear this glorious and fearful name, THE LORD THY GOD; then the Lord will make thy plagues wonderful, and the plagues of thy seed, even great plagues, and of long continuance, and sore sicknesses, and of long continuance. Moreover, he will bring upon thee all the diseases of Egypt, which thou was afraid of; and they shall cleave unto thee. Also, every sickness and every plague which is not written in the book of this law, them will the Lord bring upon thee, until thou be destroyed."

Perhaps this warning is not without merit as, apparently, blood-borne viruses were present in antiquity. The book of Leviticus, Chapter 11, appears to be a dietary prescription to avoid the possibility of transfection from a blood-born virus (such as AIDS). Leviticus 7:26 states, "Moreover ye shall eat no manner of blood, whether it be of fowl or of beast, in any of your dwellings. Whatsoever soul it be that eateth any manner of blood, even that soul shall be cutoff from his people." Leviticus 17:10 states, "And whatsoever man there be of the house of Israel, or of the strangers that sojourn among you, that eateth any manner of blood; I will even set my face against that soul that eateth blood, and will cut him off from among his people."

According to John Frazer, in *The Golden Bough,* blood taboos have been observed by other cultures throughout history:

> "Some Esthonians will not taste blood because they believe that it contains the animal's soul, which would enter the body of the person who tasted the blood. Some Indian tribes of North America through a strong principle of religion, abstain in the strictest manner from eating the blood of any animal, as it contains the life and spirit of the beast. Jewish hunters poured out the blood of the game they had killed and covered it up with dust. They would not taste the blood, believing that the soul or life of the animal was in the blood, or actually was the blood."[1]

Why this universal prohibition concerning blood? Frazer continues:

> "Among the Latuka of Central Africa the earth on which a drop of blood has fallen at childbirth is carefully scraped up with an iron shovel, put into a pot along with the water used in washing the mother, and buried tolerably deep outside the house on the left-hand side. In West Africa, if a drop of your blood has fallen on the ground, you must carefully cover it up, rub and stamp it into the soil; if it has fallen on the side of a canoe or a tree, the place is cut out and the chip destroyed."

Other primitive taboos involve blood from menstruation or childbirth. Consider Leviticus 15:19, "And if a woman have an issue, and her issue in her flesh be blood, she shall be put apart seven days: and whosoever toucheth her shall be unclean until the even and every thing that she lieth upon in her separation shall be unclean: every thing also that she sitteth upon shall be unclean." Leviticus 12:2 (380) states, "Speak unto the children of Israel, saying, if a woman have conceived seed, and born a man child: then she shall be unclean seven days." According to Frazier, aboriginal:

> "[Aboriginal] Australian women (during menstruation) are forbidden under pain of death to touch anything that men use, or even to walk on a path that any man frequents. They are also secluded at childbirth, and all vessels used by them during their seclusion are burned. In Uganda the pots which a woman touches while the impurity of childbirth or of menstruation is on her should be destroyed. Among the Bribri Indians of Costa Rica a menstrous woman is regarded as unclean. She drinks out of a special vessel because if anyone drank out of the same cup after her, (according to the Bribri) he would surely die."
>
> "In Tahiti a woman after childbirth was secluded for a fortnight or three weeks in a temporary hut erected on sacred ground—if anyone touched her or the child at this period, he was subjected to the same restrictions as the mother until the ceremony of her purification had been performed. In the island of Kodiak, off Alaska, a woman about to be delivered retires to a miserable low hovel built of reeds, where she must remain for twenty days after the birth, she is considered so unclean that no one will touch her, and food is reached to her on sticks."

Could it be that the apparent universal prohibition of contact with blood has some long-lost logical reason?

Speaking of sexual intercourse and sexual behavior among primitive peoples, Frazer states:

> "We have seen that at critical periods the life or soul is sometimes temporarily stowed away in a safe place till the danger is past. But institutions like totemism are not resorted to merely on special occassions of danger; they are systems into which everyone, or at least every male, is obliged to be initiated at a certain period of life. Now the period of life at which initiation takes place is regularly puberty; and this fact suggests that the special danger which totemism and systems like it are intended to obviate is supposed not to arise till sexual maturity has been attained, in fact, that the danger apprehended is believed to attend the relation of the sexes to each other. It would be easy to prove by a long array of facts that sexual relation is associated in the primitive mind with many serious perils; but the exact nature of the danger apprehended is still obscure. We may hope that a more exact acquaintance with savage modes of thought will in time disclose this central mystery of primitive society, and will thereby furnish the clue, not only to totemism but to the origin of the marriage system."

Regarding semen as a source of potential transfection, Leviticus 15:16 states, "And if any man's seed of copulation go out from him, then he shall wash all his flesh in water, and be unclean until the evening. And every garment, and every skin, whereon is the seed of copulation, shall be washed with water, and be unclean until the evening. The woman also with whom man shall lie with seed of copulation, they shall both bathe themselves in water, and be unclean until the evening." Did sexual relations play some role in some long-forgotten blood-borne virus epidemic?

In examination of the historical taboos across time and across cultures regarding blood and sexual irresponsiblity, a theme appears which is so universal that an argument can be advanced that the relationship of "morality" and the importance of blood in seriously devastating plagues cannot be ignored. Leviticus 13 describes the characteristics for diagnosis (called leprosy, but referring to any host of skin diseases in addition to Hansen's Disease) among the Hebrew tribes which bears striking similarity to some symptoms observed in AIDS. Among those symptoms to be observed were: a rising, scab, or bright spot on the skin; hair in the plague on the skin is white, the plague on the skin is deeper than the skin, the scab spreads in the skin, raw flesh, a yellowish thinning of the hair of the head or beard, a scale spreading in the skin, and hair falling out accompanied by weeping sores.

Finally, this view would appear to advocate that the epidemic is a result of retribution from God for failure to conform to a set of guidelines and that the major prescriptive intervention should be a return to God's stated guidelines for human relations. Because a God-based view of the epidemic should focus on change of societal behaviors rather than making a moralistic judgment of the infected individuals themselves, this view may, if consistently and truly applied, provide numbers of volunteers to support those who are infected.

Human Cause by Design

This interpretation of the AIDS epidemic has been proposed by organizations such as the Lyndon LaRoche's political party. The reader will recall in chapter one that this organization has proposed that the disease may be the result of a "grand conspiracy" of the Trilateral Commission Elite to reduce the influence of the United States as a world power so as to create an environment conducive to establishment of a "one-world system." Such an underpinning philosophy/moralizing can be particularly dangerous as the disease claims more and more lives.

Undoubtedly conspiracy theories attributing the cause of AIDS to various human agents, governments, or organizations will become more popular in the future—the result of a fearful public looking for someone/something to blame. Prescriptive interventions based on this underpinning view may include extremely radical treatment of AIDS victims, perhaps including euthanasia and, at the same time, seeking to "dethrone" the conspirators (a scapegoat) and find the "hidden antidote." This strategy would appear to preempt logical solution to the AIDS problem and create a societal mood potentially highly discriminatory to infected individuals based on emotion rather than fact.

Natural Cause by Accident

The accepted view by the scientific community at present is that through random biological processes the AIDS retrovirus mutated from the STLV-III virus and was through chance subsequently transmitted to humans from the Green Monkey somewhere in east-central Africa. This thesis, as emphasized throughout this book, appears to provide a framework for logical solution of the epidemic and promote a logical view of infected individual's rights consistent with disease transmission vectors.

Human Cause by Accident

A likely "fear of technology" based view is that science is the cause of the disease. Doubtlessly unsupported allegations of recombinant DNA (genetic manipulation) research in bio-chemical warfare development might be expected. Other "causes" may rest in the host of other environmental pollutions man has been excessively doing since the 1940s, e. g., above ground nuclear testing, herbicide usage, or indiscriminate discarding of toxic wastes. Such a view may likely hold the opinion that AIDS is a "natural" result of both national and corporate environmental irresponsibility and that the infected are victims of this irresponsibility.

Epilogue

There are many potentials for moralizing/philosophizing about AIDS some of which have been presented here. Most important is the fact that as the disease drastically spreads, underpinning views of the disease may have an impact on resultant social response to the disease.

Regarding advent of AIDS by "design" from either natural or divine agents, the historical anthropological study of taboos seems to provide a universal warning against sexual irresponsibility, the danger of blood, and the relationship of the two regardless of culture. Indeed, it appears that "morality" or the practice of responsible sexual behavior is not a "should" but, in fact, a "must" in order to avoid plague. Whether the argument of natural or divine judgement is valid is not the issue—what may be the issue is the fact that in every culture around the world and across time the responsible practice of one's sexuality has been critical to a society's survival. The historical records of cultures clearly point to irresponsible sexuality as a major factor contributing to a society's demise. From a strictly logical and historical perspective Americans must become responsible for their sexual behavior or be counted among those cultures which ignored the call to the responsible practice of their individual and national sexuality.

Regarding "conspiracy" theories as a cause for AIDS, any philosophy advocating this view will, in both the short and long term, focus necessary activity away from individuals' collective responsibility for their own sexual behavior through "witch hunting" for some conspirator. Further, the result of such a view holds that, at some point, it is necessary that a scapegoat be found—whether the victims themselves, science, government, or other groups.

With AIDS, the previous discussion not withstanding, there is a moral—in the very simplest of terms that moral is this: if you are sexually irresponsible you will die and if a nation is sexually irresponsible it dies. Whether the "cause" is by nature, God, science, or political machination, the bottom line is that sexual irresponsibility now ends in death.

Notes

[1] Leishman, K. "Heterosexuals and AIDS," *The Atlantic Monthly*, Feb. 1987: 39.

[2] Frazer, J. G., *The Golden Bough* (New York: The Macmillian Company 1923) 228.

AIDS: What Must Be Done?

Substantial evidence has been presented to prove that the AIDS epidemic is, without doubt, the most challenging problem that has ever confronted this nation. In terms of potential social upheaval, economic destruction, and loss of life, AIDS stands as a most awesome potential destructor, rivaled only by thermonuclear war. As Dr. Stephen Gould of Harvard University pointed out, AIDS has the potential to kill perhaps one-quarter of the entire human species and the possibility exists for even greater loss of life. Though that destruction will not be instantaneous, it will be relentless. Such a threat calls for action unprecedented in the history of the United States. What unprecedented action shall come is and will be predicated on basic assumptions made about the disease and its victims as well as the degree of logical anticipatory planning developed. If AIDS is perceived from a basis of fear quite different choices will be made than if AIDS is perceived as a challenging opportunity to change not only our individual and national sexual behavior but our individual and national compassion. The critical "window" of strategy choice is, even now, beginning to close, and resulting choices will no doubt have long-lasting impact on how we, as individuals and a people, regard our selves and our nation. Indeed, the choice will clearly effect our individual and collective existence.

The nation, in the interest of long-term survival, may need to consider temporary modification/suspension of some of what could be in this crisis defined as short-term privileges. Philosophically, the construction of general non-discriminatory policy within the context of short-term economic gain may be, in the longer term, irrational, despite the fact that those policies certainly have shorter-term ethical merit. However, present shorter-term strategies will soon lead to a point when moral questions will become extremely difficult and subsequent resolutions greatly polarized. Extremely simplified questions can be distilled to that of individual *vs.* the collective welfare.

Those who would argue that current non-discriminatory strategies are ethical, appear to be those who are most negatively affected economically. Those who morally defend non-discrimination are justified in doing so, but if in doing so the collective welfare of the nation is ignored then their judgement is certainly open to question. This method will surely provoke a backlash against civil liberties as the disease spreads. In fact, by their very defense of individual liberties non-discrimination advocates may be hastening the total removal of those liberties.

Of interest, in May 1987 disagreement surfaced within the U. S. administration as to how to control the spread of AIDS. Education Secretary William Bennett's Georgetown University call for mandatory AIDS testing for hospital patients, immigrants, prisoners and engaged couples applying for marriage licenses was in direct disagreement with Surgeon General Koop's and Public Health Service officials who advocate voluntary testing. Why is the Secretary of Education publicly advocating a public health policy in direct contradiction to that of the Surgeon General? Obviously, confusion within the Reagan Administration exists regarding civil liberties and AIDS as Koop continues to advocate voluntary testing while others publicly advocate mandatory testing. Mandatory testing could cost the federal government billions of dollars. Is it civil liberties, dollars, or public health that matters? Is the short term or the long term more important?

Preventing Political Backlash

A prudent approach for civil libertarians is to prevent the public's polarization on the issue of individual *vs.* collective welfare. This can be done by focusing effort on containment of the disease and avoiding or minimizing civil libertarian litigation. In so doing, longer-term economic and civil liberty interests will be maintained. To focus effort on any issue (e. g., non-discrimination) but the containment of AIDS will insure the demise of those longer-term interests from reactionary elements of a frightened society. Simply put, AIDS must be de-politicized as an issue of rights and politicized as a problem which must be contained. This will not come without grassroot political activity since both the federal government and civil libertarians appear to have short-term vested interests in preventing a realistically appropriate response to the AIDS epi
demic, i. e., money and special interests, respectively.

Political coalitions should be forged across all population groups, including the gay and heterosexual communities, as well as the legal, medical, insurance, business, and labor communities advocating the goal of disease containment with the objective of overcoming short-term perceived benefits at the eventual cost of long-term national survival. Obviously no group will benefit from the continued spread of the disease and all groups will benefit from disease containment. Those coalitions must then collectively lobby state and federal governments to develop, sanction, and assist in funding interventive strategies which would insure strong measures for disease containment. Even though past efforts to contain and/or regulate citizens' sexual behavior have not been successful, that past history does not rule out the possibility of regulation if powerful measures are instituted through grassroots political activity.

A major problem of our democratic form of government is that it cannot swiftly respond to this disease without consensus among its constituents. Currently that consensus does not exist among the scientific community or the aforementioned groups. This lack of consensus, particularly brought about within the general public as a result of a lack of scientifically validated information, is delaying a unified response to disease containment strategies at a time when each day of delay results in an additional 1,000 persons being infected by the disease. To move to consensus, in absence of strong federal leadership, it is absolutely essential that education regarding the potential impact of AIDS on the American society be provided on a wide scale. Such a demand necessitates grassroots political lobbying.

It is not all the individuals within any group that contribute to disease spread but those members in a group continuing irresponsible sexuality, thereby placing others at risk. The common ground of all political groups' coalitions is not discrimination against any group as a whole but that portion of any group which continues sexual irresponsiblity and increases risks for all groups. Public education of methods to avoid the disease must continue. We must recognize the fact that education may not be greatly effective in stopping disease spread —particularly if individuals do not know their HTLV-III/LAV status.

Strong interventive strategies for disease containment should be directed specifically toward those individuals of any group continuing irresponsible behavior. Irresponsible behavior is any behavior knowingly perpetrated by an individual which transmits the disease to a non-infected individual. The AIDS problem could and should be shifted by this approach from an issue of civil liberties to an issue of criminal conduct. All groups in a coalition directing effort toward that end will benefit and discrimination against any group other than the irresponsible will be circumvented.

A Modest Proposal?

What we should do about those individuals of any group engaging in criminally irresponsible sexual conduct is the issue. The cost of quarantine of an entire group would be prohibitive. However, as the disease remains non-communicable through casual contact, the identification and containment of criminal elements from among any group may become comparatively and fiscally possible. Cost for containment of the sexually irresponsible, when considered in light of a potential $10 trillion national medical expense if the disease goes unchecked, appears comparatively minimal but could be substantial. The argument that compulsory testing will drive those who need services underground may be true, but when compared to the magnitude of the epidemic perhaps a better argument for compulsory testing is that it would, if appropriately designed, drive those who don't know their HTLV-III/LAV status to find out. Once an individual knows their HTLV-III/LAV status then, and only then, can personal responsibility for the spread of the disease be established. Without awareness of condition an individual cannot, nor should not, be held responsible for criminal conduct.

Identification of those persons who are irresponsibly putting others at risk regardless of group can only be accomplished through active assistance of the general population. Again, consensus must exist. In order for individuals to report criminally sexually irresponsible persons, the general population must be potentially capable of determining an individual's HTLV-III/LAV status. Such an approach shall require that the general population be periodically tested for the presence of the virus.

The effort to provide an inexpensive and reliable HTLV-III/LAV blood test is currently underway and may be available within 2-5 years or sooner. On Friday, February 13, 1987, the University of California at Davis announced that it had developed a fast, easy and cheap method of screening blood samples for the

AIDS virus called the *DOT EIA*. While currently undergoing tests for validity, the *DOT EIA*, if effective, could detect individuals infected with the virus, detect AIDS-contaminated blood, and provide the ability to track the spread of the epidemic. Palmer Beasley, an internationally known epidemiologist at San Francisco General Hospital, said of the test, "if easier and cheaper [the test] means that screening could be done and it would be a relatively simple way of doing something to protect some people."[1] The *DOT EIA* is the first screening test that needs no sophisticated equipment or highly trained technicians to conduct. It is a step toward affordable testing—costing only $.25-$.30 per test compared to the ELISA's $2.00-$6.00 per test and requires only 30 minutes to perform. It does, however, require several hours of instruction before one can administer it. Once simplified this, or a similar test, should be periodically delivered to the general United States' population.

Regarding mass screening potential derived from the *DOT EIA*, the World Health Organization (WHO), however, warns that the "marketing of such tests should be approached with caution in Western nations, because their availability may encourage mass screening for the virus before the consequences of such screening are adequately explored."[2] Dr. Jonathan Mann, director of the WHO's Special Program on AIDS stated, "If we get to the point that you can test for the AIDS virus with a finger stick and a drop of blood, it may create the temptation to use screening in developed countries without full social discussion and reflection."[3] Dr. James R. Carlson, an assistant professor of pathology at University of California at Davis and leader of the research team developing the *DOT EIA* remarked, "There is no question that the technology is out there to develop a test that could be used in the home, like a pregnancy test—the issue is whether you would want to use the test in the community"[4] and there are no current plans to seek marketing approval from the U. S. Food and Drug Administration.

It is this writer's opinion that to have the means of fast, inexpensive testing and not to use it, given the unprecedented seriousness of the epidemic and its ramifications for collective American society, borders on irrationality and must be overcome. Dr. Patrick Riley, past president of the Washoe County Medical Society and a pathologist at Saint Mary's Hospital in Reno, Nevada said in 1987, "If you believe the figures coming out from the CDC—and I do—then mandatory testing is a reasonable approach."[5]

Coordination and guidance of a national testing program should ultimately become a legislated federal responsibility with delegated responsibility to states. Although individuals within states may choose to avoid testing, failure to show evidence that a test has been done would result in their loss of state privileges, e. g., vehicle license plates, driver's license, state welfare services, unemployment compensation, and other periodically reoccurring contacts between the individual and state government. Systems of verifying individuals' privileges are already in place. Making continued participation in state privileges contingent upon verification from a state's public health department that a blood test has been recently done would be a relatively inexpensive and technologically feasible systems' addition—the cost of the actual test being the citizen's responsibility. To preserve privacy of the results of an individual's blood test the actual HTLV-III/LAV status would be reported directly to each state's public health department from a designated testing site and only the fact that a test has been done would be shared with other state departments. It would be an individual's choice and responsibility to report to designated testing facilities. Once an individual's HIV status is determined potential identification by the general population of irresponsible AIDS-infected individuals becomes possible.

A Long Term Necessary Intervention?

To be truly effective, identification must be public so as to allow general population members the right and freedom to avoid infection. At the same time, however, any method of public identification must be such that a seropositive individual's status is *only* revealed during a potential high-risk activity and at no other time. This type of identification strategy would prevent general discrimination and preserve the individual's privacy while at the same time provide the general public the opportunity to avoid infection.

A method meeting both requirements could be discreet genital tattooing—just inside the urethra for males; just inside the labia minora for females—but that strategy is bound to elicit strong negative emotional reactions, summoning images of Nazi Germany. The issue of discreet genital tattooing, however, must be considered as the least restrictive, least costly, and most humane of any effective strategy for public identification of infected individuals—any alternative would be more restrictive, costly, and discriminatory. Not to allow potential identification of irresponsible individuals is to deny the general population the right to non-infection. With the rights of responsible infected individuals being maintained as the disease remains non-communicable through casual contact, the collective welfare can be protected.

Physical confinement of sexually irresponsible individuals is not economically practical. If confinement costs per year resembled current annual costs for prisoner housing ($30,000 per person per year) and the number of irresponsible sexual offenders approached 20% of the AIDS-infected population, then confine-ment costs per year as of 1987 would be $15 billion; by A. D. 2001 it could approach $300 billion. Those costs, coupled with anticipated medical and social service costs, could not be sustained. Quarantine or confinement is not the answer. However, if an individual is contributing to the spread of the disease, an alternative is to make that individual's infection status publicly visible through a highly visible tattoo—his/her quarantine within the society being accomplished through public visibility of his/her status. It is a rational consequence that if the individual cannot or will not be responsible to society then society must be capable of protecting itself.

The issue of public identification will be highly emotional and may likely result in identification of all persons infected as fear grows or if casual contact is documented as a vector in transmission, unless appropriate action is now taken. If that does occur, it will be the result of greatly increased concern about the economic implications posed for the nation and panic among non-infected individuals—both brought about from failure to logically attack this pandemic. Very likely public identification will be brought about as a "national security measure" and civil liberties of many types will be suspended. Again the compassionate approach is to maintain the responsible infected individual's right to continue in society while at the same time protecting the general population.

Resistance to testing of the general population once cheaper identification tests are released will become less defensible as the numbers of the infected increase. If public identification strategies are affected for the general population of AIDS-infected individuals, identification must be done in such a way as to absolutely maintain the individual's privacy to avoid discrimination in every situation except that for which public identification is designed, i. e., high-risk behavior contact. To avoid public identification of infected responsible individuals in situations of public nudity, e. g., public showers, placement of any discreet tattoo must be such that it is only seen when sexual contact or other high-risk behavior is considered. Other areas of the body beside the genital region may be appropriate—maintaining privacy yet visibility when sexual contact or other high-risk behavior is desired. Perhaps inside and high in the top lip of an individual on the mucous membrane would be appropriate.

As previously mentioned, this strategy is very likely to provoke extreme resistance particularly among those individuals who are not sufficiently aware of the potential destructiveness of this disease on the nation's economy and social systems. Given the wide spread of the disease, the potential economic and social impact, the inability of national systems to respond appropriately to a runaway epidemic, and the methods through which the disease is currently being transmitted, this writer challenges the reader to develop alternative, yet equally effective, strategies to maintain individual freedoms and the collective welfare. Logical attacks on the disease are paramount.

A Major Scientific Research Assault is Required

Public identification will do nothing to affect the epidemic other than to reduce the risk of the spread of AIDS and to prevent irresponsible individuals from maliciously contributing to the epidemic. At the same time that any effort is made for public identification of irresponsible individuals, there must be a national, even world, research program funded on a level surpassing any historic scientific endeavor seen to date. By comparison, funding for AIDS vaccine/cure research should be greater than that which was spent during the 1960s Apollo Moon missions; greater than that which has been spent in the last 5 years for American military rearmament ($1.5 trillion) and that level of funding must be directed toward research *now*. Larry Kessler, executive director of the AIDS Action Committee of Boston, Massachusetts stated in February 1987, "The federal government is still thinking about how to spend a few bucks here and there: this thing requires the equivalent of the whole defense budget. This is a greater threat to American than communism in Nicaragua."[6]

Very simply, if a vaccine/cure is not developed soon, federal funds for research may be reduced in the flood-tide of medical and social service expenses. Already some of the federal dollars spent on AIDS come from other programs at the National Institutes of Health, shortchanging other health needs. A very real world security problem could exist as nations may need to divert military spending to solve the AIDS epidemic. Those countries which can halt the AIDS spread in their respective country may emerge as new powers if one quarter to one half of the worlds' population is decimated.

Extensive Public Health Planning and Action Required

Finally, strategies for treatment of now-infected and soon-to-be-infected individuals must be planned. It is likely that as the number of individuals becoming sick with AIDS increases, the medical community will not be capable of providing treatment for all persons. Costs for treatment will not be affordable to a great many individuals, perhaps necessitating state or federal appropriation of AIDS victims' assets to defray costs for treatment. This probability suggests that public health services should begin now to develop neighborhood care strategies and that the staff of those programs be either volunteers, work-assigned public welfare recipients, or the working-well AIDS infected. Contingency funding strategies for these facilities should be developed to prevent more drastic funding methods. That extensive recruitment and training processes as well as alternative funding strategies be planned now and be operational by 1991 seems apparent.

Epilogue

The question "What must be done?" is one which is now provoking, and will continue to provoke, emotional reactions. The range of answers to this question run the gamut from mass testing, identification and subsequent quarantine to general public education of the urgent need to change sexual behavior. Two issues are apparently at the root of any strategy of attacking the AIDS problem. Those issues are individual *vx.* collective welfare and trust—trusting an individual to know his disease status and control his behavior or not trusting individuals and disclosing their status through some method not yet decided.

The issue of individual *vs.* collective welfare is, as of 1987, erring on the side of individual good. The issue of trust is erring on the side of an individual knowing his disease status and effectively adjusting his behavior. Both of these directions are quite noble and consistent with an idealized view of the American condition—whether that idealized view is, in reality, correct is a considerable gamble in light of the extreme effects possible from the disease. This is a particularly problematic view in light of the absence of general population AIDS testing.

In the immediate future, to forestall an emotionally-based over-reactive backlash resulting in total removal of civil liberties of infected individuals or, even worse, budget-busting quarantine/containment camps, a very blatant honesty regarding future prospects of AIDS growth in America is essential. In the absence of a mobilized effort originating among political coalitions to attack the problem, the federal government must begin development of an appropriate, discreet disease-transmission-specific public identification method. A call for testing of the general population as soon as cheaper testing methods are developed, combined with discreet genital tattooing of seropositive individuals, is one method of approaching this unprecedented challenge.

Not even remotely considered under *any* other circumstance, this approach can maximize the freedom of the responsible infected individual, maximize the visibility of the irresponsible infected individual, and maximize the welfare of the general community. While contrary to American concepts of freedom, a discreet method of public identification of individuals must be considered as a sacrifice for the longer-term preservation of American civil liberties. To argue against this approach while doing nothing to reduce the rampant spread of the disease is indefensible. At current AIDS growth rates the nation has, in a best case, 23 years to go before a major depopulation occurs. AIDS is no joke and is certain to test the nation's logic and compassion.

Notes

[1] Robinson-Haynes, E. "Fast, Cheap Test for AIDS Virus," *Sacramento (California) Bee* Feb. 14, 1987.

[2] Steinbrook, R. "Cheap, Speedy Test Found for AIDS Virus Found," *Los Angeles (California) Times* Feb. 14, 1987.

[3] Steinbrook.

[4] Steinbrook.

[5] Santich, K. "State Health Professionals See Expanded AIDS Testing," *Reno (Nevada) Gazette-Journal* Feb. 8, 1987.

[6] Howard, M. "Fund Shortage Looms as Cases on Increase," *Boston (Massachusetts) Herald* Feb. 15, 1987.

Epilogue

This book has attempted to present the AIDS epidemic in America as it *may* develop. A case has been presented using substantial documentation that the possibilities for an unprecedented challenge to each of us may lie in the near future (during the next 15-20 years) *if* an effective vaccine/cure is not soon developed.

The potential impact on the American federal government may be tremendous, affecting the government's ability to continue provision of social welfare programming in the same manner as it exists today. Change in the economy of the nation may lie ahead as the disease exponentially grows. Change in the structure of the American nuclear family may result and the potential for increased numbers of extended families living as a single unit appears possible as the nation's "security net" fails.

The potential impact on the medical profession may be equally profound. The possibility exists that the medical community as it now exists will not be capable of meeting the needs of the millions who may need services. The resulting impact on medical costs, as a function of decreased private health insurance availability, may create civil disobedience and the creation of nationalized health insurance which would place great stress on the nation's economy. Additional stress on the nation's insurance industry and business appears likely.

Efforts toward creation of vaccines and treatments for AIDS have been examined with not particularly encouraging conclusions. A case has been made that the present epidemic in America may be at least partially associated with a decline in the responsible practice of sexuality by members of this society. Further, a case has been presented that some method of discreet disease-transmission-related public identification of infected individuals may be a method to forestall greater erosion of civil liberties.

It appears that the AIDS epi-demic, as it is now unfolding in America, is without doubt, the greatest challenge that this nation has ever and may ever face. The social upheaval from a runaway epidemic may very likely result in significant changes in how this country is administered particularly when AIDS threatens to be capable of completely devastating the national economy through either a deflationary or hyperinflationary depression. This pressure, combined with either a gradual erosion or sudden backlash removal of civil liberties, strongly suggests that an authoritarian or totalitarian system of government may be a result of the challenge. It also appears possible that as this disease advances, coupled with incredible health costs and an inability of the government to support such costs, that lawlessness will increase.

The confusion created by this disease may have unpredictable geopolitical and national security consequences. If other retroviruses, e. g., HTLV-I and LAV-2, further complicate the scenario and if AIDS mutates to a point where its transmission includes vectors other than sexual contact and I. V. needle sharing, i. e., demonstrated and accepted insect vectoring or casual contact, the general population may likely panic and seek scapegoats. The potential future presented in the prologue of this book, without immediate change in citizens' sexual behavior and efficient public health action and education on a scale not seen before in the history of this country, may become truth.

Finally, this book has attempted to present a possibility that *can* occur—it is not intended to sensationalize nor is it intended to frighten you into immobility. It is intended to change your sexual behavior, if necessary. It is intended to arouse you to political action. It is intended to save your life. Educational and provocative in nature, this book may not only save your life, depending upon your responsible sexual behavior, but help save this nation.

Helpful Information

HOTLINES and related support services*

AZT Hotline at the National Institutes of Health: 1-800-843-9388; 8 A.M. to midnight (EST), seven days a week.
Baltimore, Maryland AIDS Hotline: 1-800-323-AIDS.
California Suicide Prevention Hotline #1: 1-408-649-8008.
California Suicide Prevention Hotline #2: 1-415-367-8000.
Centers for Disease Control AIDS Hotline: 1-800-342-AIDS; 24 hours, seven days a week.
Chicago DPH—AIDS Activity Office #1: 1-312- 744-4305.
Chicago DPH—AIDS Activity Office #2: 1-312-744-4306.
Civil Rights Hotline: 1-800-368-1019.
Dallas, Texas Gay Alliance AIDS Taskforce: 1-214-528-4233.
Hawaii AIDS Hotline: 1-800- 735-5303.
Hemophilia Foundation, New York, NY: 1-212- 682-5510.
Houston, Texas AIDS Hotline: 1-800-548-8378.
IV Substance Abuse-AIDS Hotline, New York, NY: 1-212-420-4141.
Los Angeles, California AIDS Hotline: 1-800-443-0810.
Los Angeles, California AIDS Project: 1-213-876-AIDS.
Miami, Florida Health Crisis Network: 1-305-326-8833.
National AIDS Hotline: 1-800-243-AIDS.
National American AIDS Hotline: 1-800-992-4379.
National Gay Taskforce Crisisline: 1-800-221-7044.
National Health Information Clearinghouse: 1-800-336-4797.
National Hepatitis Hotline: 1-800-223-0179.
National Institute of Drug Abuse Hotline: 1-800-662-HELP.
National PHS AIDS Hotline #1: 1-800-342-AIDS.
National PHS AIDS Hotline #2: 1-800-342-7514.
National Sexually Transmitted Diseases Hotline: 1-800-227-8922.

*Hotline and supportive service telephone numbers are constantly changing. This list was accurate as of July 1987.

New Orleans, Louisiana AIDS Hotline: 1-800-634-7477.
New York City Pediatrics Hotline: 1-212-430-3333.
New York City Suicide Prevention Hotline: 1-212-532-2400.
New York City Upper West Side AIDS Project: 1-800-874-5178.
Philadelphia, Pennsylvania AIDS Hotline: 1-215-732-AIDS.
Project Inform Hotline: 1-800-822-7422.
Public Health Service National AIDS Hotline: 1-800-342-AIDS.
San Diego, California AIDS Project: 1-619-260-1304.
San Francisco, California AIDS Foundation: 1-415-FOR-AIDS.

ORGANIZATIONS

1. AIDS Action Council
   Washington, DC 20003
   1-202-547-3101

2. AIDS Action Project
   Chicago, IL 60613
   1-800-243-2437

3. AIDS Coordinator
   Connecticut Department of Health
   Hartford, CT 06106
   1-203-566-5058

4. American Academy of Pediatrics
   Elk Grove Village, IL 60007
   1-312-228-5005

5. American Association of Physicians for Human Rights
   San Francisco, CA 94114
   1-415-558-9353

6. American College Health Association
   Rockville, MD 20855
   1-301-963-1100

7. American Foundation for AIDS Research
   New York, NY 10019 or Los Angeles, CA 90210-5294
   1-212-333-3118 1-213-273-5547

8. American Foundation of AIDS Research
Los Angeles, CA 90210
1-213-273-5547

9. American Public Health Association
Washington, DC 20005
1-202-789-6500

10. American Red Cross AIDS Education Program
Washington, DC 20006
1-202-639-3223; 1-292-737-8300

11. Centers for Disease Control
Atlanta, GA 30333
1-404-329-3479

12. Fenway Community Health Center
Boston, MA 02115
1-617-267-7573

13. Fund for Human Dignity
New York, NY 10012

14. Gay Men's Health Crisis
New York, NY 10011
1-212-807-7035

15. Hyacinth Foundation
Highland Park, NJ 08904
1-201-246-8439

16. KS/AIDS Foundation of Houston
Houston, TX 77006
1-713-524-2437

17. Mothers of AIDS Patients
San Diego, CA 92102
1-619-234-3432

18. National AIDS Network
Washington, DC 20003
1-202-546-2424; 1-202-347-0390

19. National Association of People with AIDS
Washington, DC 20035
1-202-483-7979

20. National Coalition of Hispanic Health and Human Services
Washington, DC 20005
1-202-371-2100

21. National Gay and Lesbian Task Force
New York, NY 10012
1-212-741-5800

22. National Institute of Allergy and Infectious Diseases
Methesda, MD 20892
1-301-496-2263

23. Shanti Foundation
West Hollywood, CA 90069
1-213-273-7591

24. For a free copy of Surgeon General C. Everett Koop's report on AIDS, write to: AIDS, Box 14252, Washington, DC 20044 or call 1-200-245-6867.

AIDS Projections by State
Assuming AIDS Distribution
Proportionate to a State's
Population.

STATE	1980 CENSUS STATE'S TOTAL POPULATION	CDC March '87 Diagnosed Cases by State (1986)	Estimated % Total Infect AIDS Populat
New York	17,558,072	10091	31.63%
California	23,667,565	7486	23.46%
Florida	9,746,324	2199	6.89%
Texas	14,229,288	2056	6.44%
New Jersey	7,364,823	1894	5.94%
Illinois	11,426,518	770	2.41%
Pennsylvania	11,863,895	708	2.22%
Massachuestts	5,737,037	678	2.12%
Georgia	5,463,105	656	2.06%
Maryland	4,216,975	509	1.60%
Washington	4,132,180	402	1.26%
Louisiana	4,206,312	395	1.24%
Conneticut	3,107,576	391	1.23%
Virginia	5,346,818	363	1.14%
Colorado	2,889,735	338	1.06%
Ohio	10,797,624	302	.95%
Michigan	9,262,078	293	.92%
Missouri	4,916,759	203	.64%
North Carolin	5,881,813	199	.62%
Arizona	2,718,425	174	.55%
Minnesota	4,075,970	172	.54%
Indiana	5,490,260	146	.46%
Oregon	2,633,149	127	.40%
Hawaii	964,691	117	.37%
South Carolin	3,121,833	114	.36%
Tennessee	4,591,120	101	.32%
Wisconsin	4,705,521	100	.31%
Oklahoma	3,025,290	99	.31%
Nevada	800,493	78	.24%
Alabama	3,893,888	75	.24%
Kentucky	3,660,257	67	.21%
Kansas	2,364,236	65	.20%
Rhode Island	947,154	63	.20%
Utah	1,461,037	59	.18%
New Mexico	1,302,981	53	.17%
Arkansas	2,286,435	51	.16%
Delaware	594,317	48	.15%
Mississippi	2,520,638	44	.14%
Iowa	2,913,808	40	.13%
Maine	1,125,027	39	.12%
New Hampshire	920,610	28	.09%
Nebraska	1,569,825	25	.08%
Alaska	401,851	25	.08%
West Virginia	1,950,279	22	.07%
Vermont	511,456	11	.03%
Idaho	944,038	8	.03%
Montana	786,690	7	.02%
Wyoming	469,557	7	.02%
South Dakota	690,768	4	.01%
North Dakota	652,717	4	.01%
	225,908,818	31906	100%

Percent of Nation's Pop. >
Now Infected this Year

Infected Total in 1987 2,182,177	Percent of State's Population Infected	Remaining Non-infected In State	Percent of Nation's Non-infected Population	State's Pop. Weighted Percent of Nation's Infected Population
690,163	4.09%	16,867,909	7.54%	15.86%
511,997	2.21%	23,155,568	10.35%	8.57%
150,398	1.57%	9,595,926	4.29%	6.08%
140,618	1.00%	14,088,670	6.30%	3.87%
129,538	1.79%	7,235,285	3.23%	6.94%
52,663	.46%	11,373,855	5.08%	1.79%
48,423	.41%	11,815,472	5.28%	1.59%
46,371	.81%	5,690,666	2.54%	3.16%
44,866	.83%	5,418,239	2.42%	3.21%
34,813	.83%	4,182,162	1.87%	3.23%
27,494	.67%	4,104,686	1.83%	2.60%
27,016	.65%	4,179,296	1.87%	2.51%
26,742	.87%	3,080,834	1.38%	3.36%
24,827	.47%	5,321,991	2.38%	1.81%
23,117	.81%	2,866,618	1.28%	3.13%
20,655	.19%	10,776,969	4.82%	.74%
20,039	.22%	9,242,039	4.13%	.84%
13,884	.28%	4,902,875	2.19%	1.10%
13,610	.23%	5,868,203	2.62%	.90%
11,901	.44%	2,706,524	1.21%	1.70%
11,764	.29%	4,064,206	1.82%	1.12%
9,986	.18%	5,480,274	2.45%	.71%
8,686	.33%	2,624,463	1.17%	1.28%
8,002	.84%	956,689	.43%	3.24%
7,797	.25%	3,114,036	1.39%	.97%
6,908	.15%	4,584,212	2.05%	.58%
6,839	.15%	4,698,682	2.10%	.56%
6,771	.22%	3,018,519	1.35%	.87%
5,335	.67%	795,158	.36%	2.60%
5,130	.13%	3,888,758	1.74%	.51%
4,582	.13%	3,655,675	1.63%	.49%
4,446	.19%	2,359,790	1.05%	.73%
4,309	.46%	942,845	.42%	1.77%
4,035	.28%	1,457,002	.65%	1.07%
3,625	.28%	1,299,356	.58%	1.08%
3,488	.15%	2,282,947	1.02%	.59%
3,283	.56%	591,034	.26%	2.15%
3,009	.12%	2,517,629	1.13%	.46%
2,736	.09%	2,911,072	1.30%	.36%
2,667	.24%	1,122,360	.50%	.92%
1,915	.21%	918,695	.41%	.81%
1,710	.11%	1,568,115	.70%	.42%
1,710	.43%	400,141	.18%	1.66%
1,505	.08%	1,948,774	.87%	.30%
752	.15%	510,704	.23%	.57%
547	.06%	943,491	.42%	.22%
479	.06%	786,211	.35%	.24%
479	.10%	469,078	.21%	.40%
274	.04%	690,494	.31%	.15%
274	.04%	652,443	.29%	.16%
2,182,177		223,726,641	100%	100%

.97%

1987 infected 2,182,177

AIDS Projections by State
Assuming AIDS Distribution
Proportionate to a State's
Population.

STATE	1980 CENSUS STATE'S TOTAL POPULATION	CDC March '87 Diagnosed Cases by State (1986)	Estimated % Total Infect AIDS Populat
New York	17,558,072	10091	31.63%
California	23,667,565	7486	23.46%
Florida	9,746,324	2199	6.89%
Texas	14,229,288	2056	6.44%
New Jersey	7,364,823	1894	5.94%
Illinois	11,426,518	770	2.41%
Pennsylvania	11,863,895	708	2.22%
Massachuestts	5,737,037	678	2.12%
Georgia	5,463,105	656	2.06%
Maryland	4,216,975	509	1.60%
Washington	4,132,180	402	1.26%
Louisiana	4,206,312	395	1.24%
Conneticut	3,107,576	391	1.23%
Virginia	5,346,818	363	1.14%
Colorado	2,889,735	338	1.06%
Ohio	10,797,624	302	.95%
Michigan	9,262,078	293	.92%
Missouri	4,916,759	203	.64%
North Carolin	5,881,813	199	.62%
Arizona	2,718,425	174	.55%
Minnesota	4,075,970	172	.54%
Indiana	5,490,260	146	.46%
Oregon	2,633,149	127	.40%
Hawaii	964,691	117	.37%
South Carolin	3,121,833	114	.36%
Tennessee	4,591,120	101	.32%
Wisconsin	4,705,521	100	.31%
Oklahoma	3,025,290	99	.31%
Nevada	800,493	78	.24%
Alabama	3,893,888	75	.24%
Kentucky	3,660,257	67	.21%
Kansas	2,364,236	65	.20%
Rhode Island	947,154	63	.20%
Utah	1,461,037	59	.18%
New Mexico	1,302,981	53	.17%
Arkansas	2,286,435	51	.16%
Delaware	594,317	48	.15%
Mississippi	2,520,638	44	.14%
Iowa	2,913,808	40	.13%
Maine	1,125,027	39	.12%
New Hampshire	920,610	28	.09%
Nebraska	1,569,825	25	.08%
Alaska	401,851	25	.08%
West Virginia	1,950,279	22	.07%
Vermont	511,456	11	.03%
Idaho	944,038	8	.03%
Montana	786,690	7	.02%
Wyoming	469,557	7	.02%
South Dakota	690,768	4	.01%
North Dakota	652,717	4	.01%
	225,908,818	31906	100%

Percent of Nation's Pop. >
Now Infected this Year

Infected Total in 1988 3,055,048	Percent of State's Population Infected	Remaining Non-infected In State	Percent of Nation's Non-infected Population	State's Pop. Weighted Percent of Nation's Infected Population
966,229	5.73%	15,901,680	7.21%	15.86%
716,796	3.10%	22,438,772	10.17%	8.57%
210,558	2.19%	9,385,368	4.25%	6.08%
196,865	1.40%	13,891,805	6.30%	3.87%
181,353	2.51%	7,053,932	3.20%	6.94%
73,729	.65%	11,300,126	5.12%	1.79%
67,792	.57%	11,747,680	5.32%	1.59%
64,920	1.14%	5,625,746	2.55%	3.16%
62,813	1.16%	5,355,426	2.43%	3.21%
48,738	1.17%	4,133,425	1.87%	3.23%
38,492	.94%	4,066,194	1.84%	2.60%
37,822	.90%	4,141,475	1.88%	2.51%
37,439	1.22%	3,043,395	1.38%	3.36%
34,758	.65%	5,287,233	2.40%	1.81%
32,364	1.13%	2,834,254	1.28%	3.13%
28,917	.27%	10,748,052	4.87%	.74%
28,055	.30%	9,213,983	4.18%	.84%
19,438	.40%	4,883,437	2.21%	1.10%
19,055	.32%	5,849,148	2.65%	.90%
16,661	.62%	2,689,864	1.22%	1.70%
16,469	.41%	4,047,737	1.83%	1.12%
13,980	.26%	5,466,295	2.48%	.71%
12,160	.46%	2,612,303	1.18%	1.28%
11,203	1.17%	945,486	.43%	3.24%
10,916	.35%	3,103,120	1.41%	.97%
9,671	.21%	4,574,541	2.07%	.58%
9,575	.20%	4,689,106	2.12%	.56%
9,479	.31%	3,009,040	1.36%	.87%
7,469	.94%	787,690	.36%	2.60%
7,181	.18%	3,881,577	1.76%	.51%
6,415	.18%	3,649,259	1.65%	.49%
6,224	.26%	2,353,567	1.07%	.73%
6,032	.64%	936,813	.42%	1.77%
5,649	.39%	1,451,352	.66%	1.07%
5,075	.39%	1,294,281	.59%	1.08%
4,883	.21%	2,278,064	1.03%	.59%
4,596	.78%	586,438	.27%	2.15%
4,213	.17%	2,513,416	1.14%	.46%
3,830	.13%	2,907,242	1.32%	.36%
3,734	.33%	1,118,625	.51%	.92%
2,681	.29%	916,014	.42%	.81%
2,394	.15%	1,565,721	.71%	.42%
2,394	.60%	397,747	.18%	1.66%
2,107	.11%	1,946,668	.88%	.30%
1,053	.21%	509,650	.23%	.57%
766	.08%	942,725	.43%	.22%
670	.09%	785,541	.36%	.24%
670	.14%	468,408	.21%	.40%
383	.06%	690,111	.31%	.15%
383	.06%	652,060	.30%	.16%
3,055,048		220,671,593	100%	100%

2.32%
1988 infected 5,237,225

AIDS Projections by State
Assuming AIDS Distribution
Proportionate to a State's
Population.

STATE	1980 CENSUS STATE'S TOTAL POPULATION	CDC March '87 Diagnosed Cases by State (1986)	Estimated % Total Infect AIDS Populat
New York	17,558,072	10091	31.63%
California	23,667,565	7486	23.46%
Florida	9,746,324	2199	6.89%
Texas	14,229,288	2056	6.44%
New Jersey	7,364,823	1894	5.94%
Illinois	11,426,518	770	2.41%
Pennsylvania	11,863,895	708	2.22%
Massachuestts	5,737,037	678	2.12%
Georgia	5,463,105	656	2.06%
Maryland	4,216,975	509	1.60%
Washington	4,132,180	402	1.26%
Louisiana	4,206,312	395	1.24%
Conneticut	3,107,576	391	1.23%
Virginia	5,346,818	363	1.14%
Colorado	2,889,735	338	1.06%
Ohio	10,797,624	302	.95%
Michigan	9,262,078	293	.92%
Missouri	4,916,759	203	.64%
North Carolin	5,881,813	199	.62%
Arizona	2,718,425	174	.55%
Minnesota	4,075,970	172	.54%
Indiana	5,490,260	146	.46%
Oregon	2,633,149	127	.40%
Hawaii	964,691	117	.37%
South Carolin	3,121,833	114	.36%
Tennessee	4,591,120	101	.32%
Wisconsin	4,705,521	100	.31%
Oklahoma	3,025,290	99	.31%
Nevada	800,493	78	.24%
Alabama	3,893,888	75	.24%
Kentucky	3,660,257	67	.21%
Kansas	2,364,236	65	.20%
Rhode Island	947,154	63	.20%
Utah	1,461,037	59	.18%
New Mexico	1,302,981	53	.17%
Arkansas	2,286,435	51	.16%
Delaware	594,317	48	.15%
Mississippi	2,520,638	44	.14%
Iowa	2,913,808	40	.13%
Maine	1,125,027	39	.12%
New Hampshire	920,610	28	.09%
Nebraska	1,569,825	25	.08%
Alaska	401,851	25	.08%
West Virginia	1,950,279	22	.07%
Vermont	511,456	11	.03%
Idaho	944,038	8	.03%
Montana	786,690	7	.02%
Wyoming	469,557	7	.02%
South Dakota	690,768	4	.01%
North Dakota	652,717	4	.01%
	225,908,818	31906	100%

Percent of Nation's Pop. >
Now Infected this Year

Infected Total in 1989 4,277,067	Percent of State's Population Infected	Remaining Non-infected In State	Percent of Nation's Non-infected Population	State's Pop. Weighted Percent of Nation's Infected Population
1,352,720	8.51%	14,548,960	6.72%	16.49%
1,003,514	4.47%	21,435,258	9.91%	8.67%
294,781	3.14%	9,090,588	4.20%	6.09%
275,611	1.98%	13,616,194	6.29%	3.85%
253,895	3.60%	6,800,037	3.14%	6.98%
103,220	.91%	11,196,906	5.17%	1.77%
94,909	.81%	11,652,771	5.38%	1.57%
90,887	1.62%	5,534,859	2.56%	3.13%
87,938	1.64%	5,267,487	2.43%	3.18%
68,233	1.65%	4,065,192	1.88%	3.20%
53,889	1.33%	4,012,305	1.85%	2.57%
52,951	1.28%	4,088,524	1.89%	2.48%
52,414	1.72%	2,990,981	1.38%	3.34%
48,661	.92%	5,238,572	2.42%	1.78%
45,310	1.60%	2,788,944	1.29%	3.10%
40,484	.38%	10,707,568	4.95%	.73%
39,277	.43%	9,174,706	4.24%	.83%
27,213	.56%	4,856,225	2.24%	1.08%
26,676	.46%	5,822,472	2.69%	.88%
23,325	.87%	2,666,539	1.23%	1.68%
23,057	.57%	4,024,680	1.86%	1.10%
19,572	.36%	5,446,723	2.52%	.69%
17,025	.65%	2,595,278	1.20%	1.26%
15,684	1.66%	929,802	.43%	3.21%
15,282	.49%	3,087,838	1.43%	.95%
13,539	.30%	4,561,002	2.11%	.57%
13,405	.29%	4,675,701	2.16%	.55%
13,271	.44%	2,995,768	1.38%	.85%
10,456	1.33%	777,234	.36%	2.57%
10,054	.26%	3,871,523	1.79%	.50%
8,981	.25%	3,640,278	1.68%	.48%
8,713	.37%	2,344,853	1.08%	.72%
8,445	.90%	928,368	.43%	1.75%
7,909	.54%	1,443,443	.67%	1.06%
7,105	.55%	1,287,177	.59%	1.06%
6,837	.30%	2,271,227	1.05%	.58%
6,435	1.10%	580,004	.27%	2.13%
5,898	.23%	2,507,517	1.16%	.45%
5,362	.18%	2,901,880	1.34%	.36%
5,228	.47%	1,113,397	.51%	.91%
3,753	.41%	912,260	.42%	.79%
3,351	.21%	1,562,370	.72%	.41%
3,351	.84%	394,396	.18%	1.63%
2,949	.15%	1,943,719	.90%	.29%
1,475	.29%	508,176	.23%	.56%
1,072	.11%	941,652	.44%	.22%
938	.12%	784,603	.36%	.23%
938	.20%	467,470	.22%	.39%
536	.08%	689,575	.32%	.15%
536	.08%	651,524	.30%	.16%
4,277,067		216,394,526	100%	100%

4.21%

1989 infected 9,514,292

AIDS Projections by State
Assuming AIDS Distribution
Proportionate to a State's
Population.

STATE	1980 CENSUS STATE'S TOTAL POPULATION	CDC March '87 Diagnosed Cases by State (1986)	Estimated % Total Infect AIDS Populat
New York	17,558,072	10091	31.63%
California	23,667,565	7486	23.46%
Florida	9,746,324	2199	6.89%
Texas	14,229,288	2056	6.44%
New Jersey	7,364,823	1894	5.94%
Illinois	11,426,518	770	2.41%
Pennsylvania	11,863,895	708	2.22%
Massachuestts	5,737,037	678	2.12%
Georgia	5,463,105	656	2.06%
Maryland	4,216,975	509	1.60%
Washington	4,132,180	402	1.26%
Louisiana	4,206,312	395	1.24%
Conneticut	3,107,576	391	1.23%
Virginia	5,346,818	363	1.14%
Colorado	2,889,735	338	1.06%
Ohio	10,797,624	302	.95%
Michigan	9,262,078	293	.92%
Missouri	4,916,759	203	.64%
North Carolin	5,881,813	199	.62%
Arizona	2,718,425	174	.55%
Minnesota	4,075,970	172	.54%
Indiana	5,490,260	146	.46%
Oregon	2,633,149	127	.40%
Hawaii	964,691	117	.37%
South Carolin	3,121,833	114	.36%
Tennessee	4,591,120	101	.32%
Wisconsin	4,705,521	100	.31%
Oklahoma	3,025,290	99	.31%
Nevada	800,493	78	.24%
Alabama	3,893,888	75	.24%
Kentucky	3,660,257	67	.21%
Kansas	2,364,236	65	.20%
Rhode Island	947,154	63	.20%
Utah	1,461,037	59	.18%
New Mexico	1,302,981	53	.17%
Arkansas	2,286,435	51	.16%
Delaware	594,317	48	.15%
Mississippi	2,520,638	44	.14%
Iowa	2,913,808	40	.13%
Maine	1,125,027	39	.12%
New Hampshire	920,610	28	.09%
Nebraska	1,569,825	25	.08%
Alaska	401,851	25	.08%
West Virginia	1,950,279	22	.07%
Vermont	511,456	11	.03%
Idaho	944,038	8	.03%
Montana	786,690	7	.02%
Wyoming	469,557	7	.02%
South Dakota	690,768	4	.01%
North Dakota	652,717	4	.01%
	225,908,818	31906	100%

Percent of Nation's Pop. >
Now Infected this Year

Infected Total in 1990 5,987,894	Percent of State's Population Infected	Remaining Non-infected In State	Percent of Nation's Non-infected Population	State's Pop. Weighted Percent of Nation's Infected Population
1,893,808	13.02%	12,655,152	6.01%	17.48%
1,404,920	6.55%	20,030,338	9.52%	8.80%
412,693	4.54%	8,677,895	4.12%	6.10%
385,856	2.83%	13,230,338	6.29%	3.81%
355,453	5.23%	6,444,584	3.06%	7.02%
144,508	1.29%	11,052,398	5.25%	1.73%
132,872	1.14%	11,519,899	5.48%	1.53%
127,242	2.30%	5,407,617	2.57%	3.09%
123,113	2.34%	5,144,374	2.44%	3.14%
95,526	2.35%	3,969,667	1.89%	3.16%
75,445	1.88%	3,936,860	1.87%	2.53%
74,131	1.81%	4,014,393	1.91%	2.43%
73,380	2.45%	2,917,601	1.39%	3.29%
68,125	1.30%	5,170,447	2.46%	1.75%
63,433	2.27%	2,725,511	1.30%	3.05%
56,677	.53%	10,650,891	5.06%	.71%
54,988	.60%	9,119,718	4.33%	.80%
38,098	.78%	4,818,127	2.29%	1.05%
37,347	.64%	5,785,125	2.75%	.86%
32,655	1.22%	2,633,884	1.25%	1.64%
32,280	.80%	3,992,400	1.90%	1.08%
27,400	.50%	5,419,323	2.58%	.68%
23,834	.92%	2,571,443	1.22%	1.23%
21,958	2.36%	907,844	.43%	3.17%
21,395	.69%	3,066,444	1.46%	.93%
18,955	.42%	4,542,047	2.16%	.56%
18,767	.40%	4,656,934	2.21%	.54%
18,580	.62%	2,977,189	1.41%	.83%
14,638	1.88%	762,595	.36%	2.53%
14,075	.36%	3,857,448	1.83%	.49%
12,574	.35%	3,627,704	1.72%	.46%
12,199	.52%	2,332,654	1.11%	.70%
11,823	1.27%	916,544	.44%	1.71%
11,073	.77%	1,432,371	.68%	1.03%
9,947	.77%	1,277,230	.61%	1.04%
9,571	.42%	2,261,656	1.07%	.57%
9,008	1.55%	570,995	.27%	2.09%
8,258	.33%	2,499,260	1.19%	.44%
7,507	.26%	2,894,373	1.38%	.35%
7,319	.66%	1,106,078	.53%	.88%
5,255	.58%	907,006	.43%	.77%
4,692	.30%	1,557,678	.74%	.40%
4,692	1.19%	389,704	.19%	1.60%
4,129	.21%	1,939,590	.92%	.29%
2,064	.41%	506,111	.24%	.55%
1,501	.16%	940,151	.45%	.21%
1,314	.17%	783,289	.37%	.22%
1,314	.28%	466,156	.22%	.38%
751	.11%	688,825	.33%	.15%
751	.12%	650,774	.31%	.15%
5,987,894		210,406,632	100%	100%

6.86%
1990 infected 15,502,186

AIDS Projections by State
Assuming AIDS Distribution
Proportionate to a State's
Population.

STATE	1980 CENSUS STATE'S TOTAL POPULATION	CDC March '87 Diagnosed Cases by State (1986)	Estimated % Total Infect AIDS Populat
New York	17,558,072	10091	31.63%
California	23,667,565	7486	23.46%
Florida	9,746,324	2199	6.89%
Texas	14,229,288	2056	6.44%
New Jersey	7,364,823	1894	5.94%
Illinois	11,426,518	770	2.41%
Pennsylvania	11,863,895	708	2.22%
Massachuestts	5,737,037	678	2.12%
Georgia	5,463,105	656	2.06%
Maryland	4,216,975	509	1.60%
Washington	4,132,180	402	1.26%
Louisiana	4,206,312	395	1.24%
Conneticut	3,107,576	391	1.23%
Virginia	5,346,818	363	1.14%
Colorado	2,889,735	338	1.06%
Ohio	10,797,624	302	.95%
Michigan	9,262,078	293	.92%
Missouri	4,916,759	203	.64%
North Carolin	5,881,813	199	.62%
Arizona	2,718,425	174	.55%
Minnesota	4,075,970	172	.54%
Indiana	5,490,260	146	.46%
Oregon	2,633,149	127	.40%
Hawaii	964,691	117	.37%
South Carolin	3,121,833	114	.36%
Tennessee	4,591,120	101	.32%
Wisconsin	4,705,521	100	.31%
Oklahoma	3,025,290	99	.31%
Nevada	800,493	78	.24%
Alabama	3,893,888	75	.24%
Kentucky	3,660,257	67	.21%
Kansas	2,364,236	65	.20%
Rhode Island	947,154	63	.20%
Utah	1,461,037	59	.18%
New Mexico	1,302,981	53	.17%
Arkansas	2,286,435	51	.16%
Delaware	594,317	48	.15%
Mississippi	2,520,638	44	.14%
Iowa	2,913,808	40	.13%
Maine	1,125,027	39	.12%
New Hampshire	920,610	28	.09%
Nebraska	1,569,825	25	.08%
Alaska	401,851	25	.08%
West Virginia	1,950,279	22	.07%
Vermont	511,456	11	.03%
Idaho	944,038	8	.03%
Montana	786,690	7	.02%
Wyoming	469,557	7	.02%
South Dakota	690,768	4	.01%
North Dakota	652,717	4	.01%
	225,908,818	31906	100%

Percent of Nation's Pop. >
Now Infected this Year

Infected Total in 1991 8,383,051	Percent of State's Population Infected	Remaining Non-infected In State	Percent of Nation's Non-infected Population	State's Pop. Weighted Percent of Nation's Infected Population
2,651,331	20.95%	10,003,821	4.95%	19.16%
1,966,888	9.82%	18,063,450	8.94%	8.98%
577,770	6.66%	8,100,125	4.01%	6.09%
540,198	4.08%	12,690,140	6.28%	3.73%
497,634	7.72%	5,946,951	2.94%	7.06%
202,311	1.83%	10,850,086	5.37%	1.67%
186,021	1.61%	11,333,877	5.61%	1.48%
178,139	3.29%	5,229,478	2.59%	3.01%
172,359	3.35%	4,972,015	2.46%	3.06%
133,736	3.37%	3,835,931	1.90%	3.08%
105,622	2.68%	3,831,238	1.90%	2.45%
103,783	2.59%	3,910,610	1.94%	2.36%
102,732	3.52%	2,814,868	1.39%	3.22%
95,375	1.84%	5,075,072	2.51%	1.69%
88,807	3.26%	2,636,704	1.31%	2.98%
79,348	.74%	10,571,543	5.23%	.68%
76,983	.84%	9,042,734	4.48%	.77%
53,337	1.11%	4,764,791	2.36%	1.01%
52,286	.90%	5,732,839	2.84%	.83%
45,717	1.74%	2,588,166	1.28%	1.59%
45,192	1.13%	3,947,209	1.95%	1.04%
38,360	.71%	5,380,963	2.66%	.65%
33,368	1.30%	2,538,075	1.26%	1.19%
30,741	3.39%	877,103	.43%	3.10%
29,953	.98%	3,036,491	1.50%	.89%
26,537	.58%	4,515,510	2.24%	.53%
26,274	.56%	4,630,660	2.29%	.52%
26,011	.87%	2,951,177	1.46%	.80%
20,494	2.69%	742,101	.37%	2.46%
19,706	.51%	3,837,742	1.90%	.47%
17,604	.49%	3,610,100	1.79%	.44%
17,078	.73%	2,315,576	1.15%	.67%
16,553	1.81%	899,991	.45%	1.65%
15,502	1.08%	1,416,869	.70%	.99%
13,925	1.09%	1,263,305	.63%	1.00%
13,400	.59%	2,248,256	1.11%	.54%
12,612	2.21%	558,384	.28%	2.02%
11,561	.46%	2,487,699	1.23%	.42%
10,510	.36%	2,883,863	1.43%	.33%
10,247	.93%	1,095,831	.54%	.85%
7,357	.81%	899,649	.45%	.74%
6,569	.42%	1,551,110	.77%	.39%
6,569	1.69%	383,136	.19%	1.54%
5,780	.30%	1,933,810	.96%	.27%
2,890	.57%	503,221	.25%	.52%
2,102	.22%	938,049	.46%	.20%
1,839	.23%	781,450	.39%	.21%
1,839	.39%	464,317	.23%	.36%
1,051	.15%	687,774	.34%	.14%
1,051	.16%	649,723	.32%	.15%
8,383,051		202,023,581	100%	100%

10.57%
1991 infected 23,885,237

AIDS Projections by State
Assuming AIDS Distribution
Proportionate to a State's
Population.

STATE	1980 CENSUS STATE'S TOTAL POPULATION	CDC March '87 Diagnosed Cases by State (1986)	Estimated % Total Infect AIDS Populat
New York	17,558,072	10091	31.63%
California	23,667,565	7486	23.46%
Florida	9,746,324	2199	6.89%
Texas	14,229,288	2056	6.44%
New Jersey	7,364,823	1894	5.94%
Illinois	11,426,518	770	2.41%
Pennsylvania	11,863,895	708	2.22%
Massachuestts	5,737,037	678	2.12%
Georgia	5,463,105	656	2.06%
Maryland	4,216,975	509	1.60%
Washington	4,132,180	402	1.26%
Louisiana	4,206,312	395	1.24%
Conneticut	3,107,576	391	1.23%
Virginia	5,346,818	363	1.14%
Colorado	2,889,735	338	1.06%
Ohio	10,797,624	302	.95%
Michigan	9,262,078	293	.92%
Missouri	4,916,759	203	.64%
North Carolin	5,881,813	199	.62%
Arizona	2,718,425	174	.55%
Minnesota	4,075,970	172	.54%
Indiana	5,490,260	146	.46%
Oregon	2,633,149	127	.40%
Hawaii	964,691	117	.37%
South Carolin	3,121,833	114	.36%
Tennessee	4,591,120	101	.32%
Wisconsin	4,705,521	100	.31%
Oklahoma	3,025,290	99	.31%
Nevada	800,493	78	.24%
Alabama	3,893,888	75	.24%
Kentucky	3,660,257	67	.21%
Kansas	2,364,236	65	.20%
Rhode Island	947,154	63	.20%
Utah	1,461,037	59	.18%
New Mexico	1,302,981	53	.17%
Arkansas	2,286,435	51	.16%
Delaware	594,317	48	.15%
Mississippi	2,520,638	44	.14%
Iowa	2,913,808	40	.13%
Maine	1,125,027	39	.12%
New Hampshire	920,610	28	.09%
Nebraska	1,569,825	25	.08%
Alaska	401,851	25	.08%
West Virginia	1,950,279	22	.07%
Vermont	511,456	11	.03%
Idaho	944,038	8	.03%
Montana	786,690	7	.02%
Wyoming	469,557	7	.02%
South Dakota	690,768	4	.01%
North Dakota	652,717	4	.01%
	225,908,818	31906	100%

Percent of Nation's Pop. >
Now Infected this Year

Infected Total in 1992 11,736,272	Percent of State's Population Infected	Remaining Non-infected In State	Percent of Nation's Non-infected Population	State's Pop. Weighted Percent of Nation's Infected Population
3,711,864	37.10%	6,291,958	3.31%	22.35%
2,753,643	15.24%	15,309,807	8.05%	9.18%
808,878	9.99%	7,291,247	3.83%	6.02%
756,277	5.96%	11,933,863	6.27%	3.59%
696,687	11.72%	5,250,263	2.76%	7.06%
283,236	2.61%	10,566,850	5.55%	1.57%
260,430	2.30%	11,073,447	5.82%	1.38%
249,395	4.77%	4,980,083	2.62%	2.87%
241,302	4.85%	4,730,713	2.49%	2.92%
187,230	4.88%	3,648,701	1.92%	2.94%
147,871	3.86%	3,683,366	1.94%	2.32%
145,296	3.72%	3,765,314	1.98%	2.24%
143,825	5.11%	2,671,043	1.40%	3.08%
133,526	2.63%	4,941,546	2.60%	1.58%
124,330	4.72%	2,512,374	1.32%	2.84%
111,087	1.05%	10,460,456	5.50%	.63%
107,777	1.19%	8,934,958	4.70%	.72%
74,671	1.57%	4,690,119	2.46%	.94%
73,200	1.28%	5,659,639	2.97%	.77%
64,004	2.47%	2,524,162	1.33%	1.49%
63,268	1.60%	3,883,940	2.04%	.97%
53,704	1.00%	5,327,258	2.80%	.60%
46,716	1.84%	2,491,360	1.31%	1.11%
43,037	4.91%	834,066	.44%	2.96%
41,934	1.38%	2,994,558	1.57%	.83%
37,152	.82%	4,478,358	2.35%	.50%
36,784	.79%	4,593,876	2.41%	.48%
36,416	1.23%	2,914,761	1.53%	.74%
28,691	3.87%	713,410	.37%	2.33%
27,588	.72%	3,810,154	2.00%	.43%
24,645	.68%	3,585,455	1.88%	.41%
23,910	1.03%	2,291,667	1.20%	.62%
23,174	2.57%	876,818	.46%	1.55%
21,703	1.53%	1,395,166	.73%	.92%
19,495	1.54%	1,243,809	.65%	.93%
18,760	.83%	2,229,496	1.17%	.50%
17,656	3.16%	540,727	.28%	1.90%
16,185	.65%	2,471,514	1.30%	.39%
14,714	.51%	2,869,150	1.51%	.31%
14,346	1.31%	1,081,485	.57%	.79%
10,299	1.14%	889,349	.47%	.69%
9,196	.59%	1,541,914	.81%	.36%
9,196	2.40%	373,940	.20%	1.45%
8,092	.42%	1,925,717	1.01%	.25%
4,046	.80%	499,175	.26%	.48%
2,943	.31%	935,106	.49%	.19%
2,575	.33%	778,875	.41%	.20%
2,575	.55%	461,742	.24%	.33%
1,471	.21%	686,302	.36%	.13%
1,471	.23%	648,251	.34%	.14%
11,736,272		190,287,309	100%	100%

15.77%
1992 infected 35,621,509

AIDS Projections by State
Assuming AIDS Distribution
Proportionate to a State's
Population.

STATE	1980 CENSUS STATE'S TOTAL POPULATION	CDC March '87 Diagnosed Cases by State (1986)	Estimated % Total Infect AIDS Populat
New York	17,558,072	10091	31.63%
California	23,667,565	7486	23.46%
Florida	9,746,324	2199	6.89%
Texas	14,229,288	2056	6.44%
New Jersey	7,364,823	1894	5.94%
Illinois	11,426,518	770	2.41%
Pennsylvania	11,863,895	708	2.22%
Massachuestts	5,737,037	678	2.12%
Georgia	5,463,105	656	2.06%
Maryland	4,216,975	509	1.60%
Washington	4,132,180	402	1.26%
Louisiana	4,206,312	395	1.24%
Conneticut	3,107,576	391	1.23%
Virginia	5,346,818	363	1.14%
Colorado	2,889,735	338	1.06%
Ohio	10,797,624	302	.95%
Michigan	9,262,078	293	.92%
Missouri	4,916,759	203	.64%
North Carolin	5,881,813	199	.62%
Arizona	2,718,425	174	.55%
Minnesota	4,075,970	172	.54%
Indiana	5,490,260	146	.46%
Oregon	2,633,149	127	.40%
Hawaii	964,691	117	.37%
South Carolin	3,121,833	114	.36%
Tennessee	4,591,120	101	.32%
Wisconsin	4,705,521	100	.31%
Oklahoma	3,025,290	99	.31%
Nevada	800,493	78	.24%
Alabama	3,893,888	75	.24%
Kentucky	3,660,257	67	.21%
Kansas	2,364,236	65	.20%
Rhode Island	947,154	63	.20%
Utah	1,461,037	59	.18%
New Mexico	1,302,981	53	.17%
Arkansas	2,286,435	51	.16%
Delaware	594,317	48	.15%
Mississippi	2,520,638	44	.14%
Iowa	2,913,808	40	.13%
Maine	1,125,027	39	.12%
New Hampshire	920,610	28	.09%
Nebraska	1,569,825	25	.08%
Alaska	401,851	25	.08%
West Virginia	1,950,279	22	.07%
Vermont	511,456	11	.03%
Idaho	944,038	8	.03%
Montana	786,690	7	.02%
Wyoming	469,557	7	.02%
South Dakota	690,768	4	.01%
North Dakota	652,717	4	.01%
	225,908,818	31906	100%

Percent of Nation's Pop. >
Now Infected this Year

Infected Total in 1993 16,430,781	Percent of State's Population Infected	Remaining Non-infected In State	Percent of Nation's Non-infected Population	State's Pop. Weighted Percent of Nation's Infected Population
5,196,609	82.59%	1,095,348	.63%	30.03%
3,855,100	25.18%	11,454,707	6.59%	9.16%
1,132,429	15.53%	6,158,817	3.54%	5.65%
1,058,788	8.87%	10,875,075	6.26%	3.23%
975,362	18.58%	4,274,901	2.46%	6.76%
396,530	3.75%	10,170,320	5.85%	1.36%
364,602	3.29%	10,708,845	6.16%	1.20%
349,153	7.01%	4,630,930	2.66%	2.55%
337,823	7.14%	4,392,889	2.53%	2.60%
262,122	7.18%	3,386,579	1.95%	2.61%
207,020	5.62%	3,476,347	2.00%	2.04%
203,415	5.40%	3,561,899	2.05%	1.96%
201,355	7.54%	2,469,688	1.42%	2.74%
186,936	3.78%	4,754,610	2.73%	1.38%
174,061	6.93%	2,338,313	1.34%	2.52%
155,522	1.49%	10,304,933	5.93%	.54%
150,888	1.69%	8,784,070	5.05%	.61%
104,540	2.23%	4,585,579	2.64%	.81%
102,480	1.81%	5,557,159	3.20%	.66%
89,606	3.55%	2,434,557	1.40%	1.29%
88,576	2.28%	3,795,365	2.18%	.83%
75,186	1.41%	5,252,072	3.02%	.51%
65,402	2.63%	2,425,958	1.40%	.95%
60,252	7.22%	773,814	.45%	2.63%
58,707	1.96%	2,935,850	1.69%	.71%
52,012	1.16%	4,426,346	2.55%	.42%
51,497	1.12%	4,542,378	2.61%	.41%
50,982	1.75%	2,863,779	1.65%	.64%
40,168	5.63%	673,242	.39%	2.05%
38,623	1.01%	3,771,531	2.17%	.37%
34,503	.96%	3,550,951	2.04%	.35%
33,473	1.46%	2,258,193	1.30%	.53%
32,443	3.70%	844,374	.49%	1.35%
30,384	2.18%	1,364,783	.79%	.79%
27,294	2.19%	1,216,515	.70%	.80%
26,264	1.18%	2,203,232	1.27%	.43%
24,719	4.57%	516,009	.30%	1.66%
22,659	.92%	2,448,855	1.41%	.33%
20,599	.72%	2,848,551	1.64%	.26%
20,084	1.86%	1,061,401	.61%	.68%
14,419	1.62%	874,930	.50%	.59%
12,874	.83%	1,529,039	.88%	.30%
12,874	3.44%	361,065	.21%	1.25%
11,329	.59%	1,914,388	1.10%	.21%
5,665	1.13%	493,510	.28%	.41%
4,120	.44%	930,987	.54%	.16%
3,605	.46%	775,270	.45%	.17%
3,605	.78%	458,137	.26%	.28%
2,060	.30%	684,242	.39%	.11%
2,060	.32%	646,191	.37%	.12%
16,430,781		173,856,528	100%	100%

23.04%
1993 infected 52,052,290

AIDS Projections by State
Assuming AIDS Distribution
Proportionate to a State's
Population.

STATE	1980 CENSUS STATE'S TOTAL POPULATION	CDC March '87 Diagnosed Cases by State (1986)	Estimated % Total Infect AIDS Populat
New York	17,558,072	10091	31.63%
California	23,667,565	7486	23.46%
Florida	9,746,324	2199	6.89%
Texas	14,229,288	2056	6.44%
New Jersey	7,364,823	1894	5.94%
Illinois	11,426,518	770	2.41%
Pennsylvania	11,863,895	708	2.22%
Massachuestts	5,737,037	678	2.12%
Georgia	5,463,105	656	2.06%
Maryland	4,216,975	509	1.60%
Washington	4,132,180	402	1.26%
Louisiana	4,206,312	395	1.24%
Conneticut	3,107,576	391	1.23%
Virginia	5,346,818	363	1.14%
Colorado	2,889,735	338	1.06%
Ohio	10,797,624	302	.95%
Michigan	9,262,078	293	.92%
Missouri	4,916,759	203	.64%
North Carolin	5,881,813	199	.62%
Arizona	2,718,425	174	.55%
Minnesota	4,075,970	172	.54%
Indiana	5,490,260	146	.46%
Oregon	2,633,149	127	.40%
Hawaii	964,691	117	.37%
South Carolin	3,121,833	114	.36%
Tennessee	4,591,120	101	.32%
Wisconsin	4,705,521	100	.31%
Oklahoma	3,025,290	99	.31%
Nevada	800,493	78	.24%
Alabama	3,893,888	75	.24%
Kentucky	3,660,257	67	.21%
Kansas	2,364,236	65	.20%
Rhode Island	947,154	63	.20%
Utah	1,461,037	59	.18%
New Mexico	1,302,981	53	.17%
Arkansas	2,286,435	51	.16%
Delaware	594,317	48	.15%
Mississippi	2,520,638	44	.14%
Iowa	2,913,808	40	.13%
Maine	1,125,027	39	.12%
New Hampshire	920,610	28	.09%
Nebraska	1,569,825	25	.08%
Alaska	401,851	25	.08%
West Virginia	1,950,279	22	.07%
Vermont	511,456	11	.03%
Idaho	944,038	8	.03%
Montana	786,690	7	.02%
Wyoming	469,557	7	.02%
South Dakota	690,768	4	.01%
North Dakota	652,717	4	.01%
	225,908,818	31906	100%

Percent of Nation's Pop. >
Now Infected this Year

Infected Total in 1994 23,003,093	Percent of State's Population Infected	Remaining Non-infected In State	Percent of Nation's Non-infected Population	State's Pop. Weighted Percent of Nation's Infected Population
7,275,253	100.00%	0	.00%	24.95%
5,397,140	47.12%	6,057,567	3.86%	11.76%
1,585,401	25.74%	4,573,416	2.91%	6.42%
1,482,303	13.63%	9,392,772	5.98%	3.40%
1,365,507	31.94%	2,909,395	1.85%	7.97%
555,143	5.46%	9,615,177	6.12%	1.36%
510,443	4.77%	10,198,402	6.49%	1.19%
488,814	10.56%	4,142,116	2.64%	2.63%
472,953	10.77%	3,919,937	2.50%	2.69%
366,971	10.84%	3,019,608	1.92%	2.70%
289,828	8.34%	3,186,519	2.03%	2.08%
284,781	8.00%	3,277,118	2.09%	2.00%
281,897	11.41%	2,187,791	1.39%	2.85%
261,710	5.50%	4,492,900	2.86%	1.37%
243,686	10.42%	2,094,627	1.33%	2.60%
217,731	2.11%	10,087,202	6.42%	.53%
211,243	2.40%	8,572,827	5.46%	.60%
146,356	3.19%	4,439,224	2.83%	.80%
143,472	2.58%	5,413,687	3.45%	.64%
125,448	5.15%	2,309,109	1.47%	1.29%
124,006	3.27%	3,671,359	2.34%	.82%
105,261	2.00%	5,146,811	3.28%	.50%
91,562	3.77%	2,334,395	1.49%	.94%
84,353	10.90%	689,461	.44%	2.72%
82,190	2.80%	2,853,660	1.82%	.70%
72,817	1.65%	4,353,529	2.77%	.41%
72,096	1.59%	4,470,282	2.85%	.40%
71,375	2.49%	2,792,403	1.78%	.62%
56,235	8.35%	617,007	.39%	2.08%
54,072	1.43%	3,717,459	2.37%	.36%
48,305	1.36%	3,502,647	2.23%	.34%
46,863	2.08%	2,211,331	1.41%	.52%
45,421	5.38%	798,953	.51%	1.34%
42,537	3.12%	1,322,246	.84%	.78%
38,211	3.14%	1,178,304	.75%	.78%
36,769	1.67%	2,166,463	1.38%	.42%
34,606	6.71%	481,402	.31%	1.67%
31,722	1.30%	2,417,133	1.54%	.32%
28,839	1.01%	2,819,712	1.80%	.25%
28,118	2.65%	1,033,284	.66%	.66%
20,187	2.31%	854,743	.54%	.58%
18,024	1.18%	1,511,015	.96%	.29%
18,024	4.99%	343,041	.22%	1.25%
15,861	.83%	1,898,526	1.21%	.21%
7,931	1.61%	485,580	.31%	.40%
5,768	.62%	925,219	.59%	.15%
5,047	.65%	770,223	.49%	.16%
5,047	1.10%	453,090	.29%	.27%
2,884	.42%	681,358	.43%	.11%
2,884	.45%	643,307	.41%	.11%
23,003,093		157,033,339	100%	100%

30.49%

1994 infected 68,875,479

AIDS Projections by State
Assuming AIDS Distribution
Proportionate to a State's
Population.

STATE	1980 CENSUS STATE'S TOTAL POPULATION	CDC March '87 Diagnosed Cases by State (1986)	Estimated % Total Infect AIDS Populat
New York	17,558,072	10091	31.63%
California	23,667,565	7486	23.46%
Florida	9,746,324	2199	6.89%
Texas	14,229,288	2056	6.44%
New Jersey	7,364,823	1894	5.94%
Illinois	11,426,518	770	2.41%
Pennsylvania	11,863,895	708	2.22%
Massachuesttts	5,737,037	678	2.12%
Georgia	5,463,105	656	2.06%
Maryland	4,216,975	509	1.60%
Washington	4,132,180	402	1.26%
Louisiana	4,206,312	395	1.24%
Conneticut	3,107,576	391	1.23%
Virginia	5,346,818	363	1.14%
Colorado	2,889,735	338	1.06%
Ohio	10,797,624	302	.95%
Michigan	9,262,078	293	.92%
Missouri	4,916,759	203	.64%
North Carolin	5,881,813	199	.62%
Arizona	2,718,425	174	.55%
Minnesota	4,075,970	172	.54%
Indiana	5,490,260	146	.46%
Oregon	2,633,149	127	.40%
Hawaii	964,691	117	.37%
South Carolin	3,121,833	114	.36%
Tennessee	4,591,120	101	.32%
Wisconsin	4,705,521	100	.31%
Oklahoma	3,025,290	99	.31%
Nevada	800,493	78	.24%
Alabama	3,893,888	75	.24%
Kentucky	3,660,257	67	.21%
Kansas	2,364,236	65	.20%
Rhode Island	947,154	63	.20%
Utah	1,461,037	59	.18%
New Mexico	1,302,981	53	.17%
Arkansas	2,286,435	51	.16%
Delaware	594,317	48	.15%
Mississippi	2,520,638	44	.14%
Iowa	2,913,808	40	.13%
Maine	1,125,027	39	.12%
New Hampshire	920,610	28	.09%
Nebraska	1,569,825	25	.08%
Alaska	401,851	25	.08%
West Virginia	1,950,279	22	.07%
Vermont	511,456	11	.03%
Idaho	944,038	8	.03%
Montana	786,690	7	.02%
Wyoming	469,557	7	.02%
South Dakota	690,768	4	.01%
North Dakota	652,717	4	.01%
	225,908,818	31906	100%

Percent of Nation's Pop. >
Now Infected this Year

Infected Total in 1995 32,204,331	Percent of State's Population Infected	Remaining Non-infected In State	Percent of Nation's Non-infected Population	State's Pop. Weighted Percent of Nation's Infected Population
0	100.00%	0	.00%	16.38%
7,555,996	100.00%	0	.00%	16.38%
2,219,561	48.53%	2,353,855	1.72%	7.95%
2,075,224	22.09%	7,317,548	5.36%	3.62%
1,911,709	65.71%	997,685	.73%	10.76%
777,200	8.08%	8,837,977	6.47%	1.32%
714,620	7.01%	9,483,782	6.95%	1.15%
684,340	16.52%	3,457,776	2.53%	2.71%
662,134	16.89%	3,257,803	2.39%	2.77%
513,759	17.01%	2,505,849	1.84%	2.79%
405,759	12.73%	2,780,760	2.04%	2.09%
398,693	12.17%	2,878,424	2.11%	1.99%
394,656	18.04%	1,793,135	1.31%	2.95%
366,394	8.15%	4,126,506	3.02%	1.34%
341,160	16.29%	1,753,466	1.28%	2.67%
304,824	3.02%	9,782,378	7.17%	.49%
295,740	3.45%	8,277,088	6.06%	.56%
204,898	4.62%	4,234,326	3.10%	.76%
200,861	3.71%	5,212,827	3.82%	.61%
175,627	7.61%	2,133,482	1.56%	1.25%
173,608	4.73%	3,497,751	2.56%	.77%
147,365	2.86%	4,999,446	3.66%	.47%
128,187	5.49%	2,206,208	1.62%	.90%
118,094	17.13%	571,367	.42%	2.81%
115,066	4.03%	2,738,595	2.01%	.66%
101,944	2.34%	4,251,584	3.11%	.38%
100,935	2.26%	4,369,347	3.20%	.37%
99,926	3.58%	2,692,478	1.97%	.59%
78,729	12.76%	538,277	.39%	2.09%
75,701	2.04%	3,641,757	2.67%	.33%
67,626	1.93%	3,435,020	2.52%	.32%
65,608	2.97%	2,145,723	1.57%	.49%
63,589	7.96%	735,364	.54%	1.30%
59,552	4.50%	1,262,694	.92%	.74%
53,496	4.54%	1,124,809	.82%	.74%
51,477	2.38%	2,114,986	1.55%	.39%
48,449	10.06%	432,953	.32%	1.65%
44,411	1.84%	2,372,721	1.74%	.30%
40,374	1.43%	2,779,338	2.04%	.23%
39,365	3.81%	993,919	.73%	.62%
28,262	3.31%	826,481	.61%	.54%
25,234	1.67%	1,485,781	1.09%	.27%
25,234	7.36%	317,807	.23%	1.20%
22,206	1.17%	1,876,321	1.37%	.19%
11,103	2.29%	474,477	.35%	.37%
8,075	.87%	917,144	.67%	.14%
7,065	.92%	763,158	.56%	.15%
7,065	1.56%	446,025	.33%	.26%
4,037	.59%	677,321	.50%	.10%
4,037	.63%	639,270	.47%	.10%
22,018,977		136,512,792	100%	100%

39.57%
1995 infected 89,396,026

AIDS Projections by State
Assuming AIDS Distribution
Proportionate to a State's
Population.

STATE	1980 CENSUS STATE'S TOTAL POPULATION	CDC March '87 Diagnosed Cases by State (1986)	Estimated % Total Infect AIDS Populat
New York	17,558,072	10091	31.63%
California	23,667,565	7486	23.46%
Florida	9,746,324	2199	6.89%
Texas	14,229,288	2056	6.44%
New Jersey	7,364,823	1894	5.94%
Illinois	11,426,518	770	2.41%
Pennsylvania	11,863,895	708	2.22%
Massachuestts	5,737,037	678	2.12%
Georgia	5,463,105	656	2.06%
Maryland	4,216,975	509	1.60%
Washington	4,132,180	402	1.26%
Louisiana	4,206,312	395	1.24%
Conneticut	3,107,576	391	1.23%
Virginia	5,346,818	363	1.14%
Colorado	2,889,735	338	1.06%
Ohio	10,797,624	302	.95%
Michigan	9,262,078	293	.92%
Missouri	4,916,759	203	.64%
North Carolin	5,881,813	199	.62%
Arizona	2,718,425	174	.55%
Minnesota	4,075,970	172	.54%
Indiana	5,490,260	146	.46%
Oregon	2,633,149	127	.40%
Hawaii	964,691	117	.37%
South Carolin	3,121,833	114	.36%
Tennessee	4,591,120	101	.32%
Wisconsin	4,705,521	100	.31%
Oklahoma	3,025,290	99	.31%
Nevada	800,493	78	.24%
Alabama	3,893,888	75	.24%
Kentucky	3,660,257	67	.21%
Kansas	2,364,236	65	.20%
Rhode Island	947,154	63	.20%
Utah	1,461,037	59	.18%
New Mexico	1,302,981	53	.17%
Arkansas	2,286,435	51	.16%
Delaware	594,317	48	.15%
Mississippi	2,520,638	44	.14%
Iowa	2,913,808	40	.13%
Maine	1,125,027	39	.12%
New Hampshire	920,610	28	.09%
Nebraska	1,569,825	25	.08%
Alaska	401,851	25	.08%
West Virginia	1,950,279	22	.07%
Vermont	511,456	11	.03%
Idaho	944,038	8	.03%
Montana	786,690	7	.02%
Wyoming	469,557	7	.02%
South Dakota	690,768	4	.01%
North Dakota	652,717	4	.01%
	225,908,818	31906	100%

Percent of Nation's Pop. >
Now Infected this Year

Infected Total in 1996 45,086,063	Percent of State's Population Infected	Remaining Non-infected In State	Percent of Nation's Non-infected Population	State's Pop. Weighted Percent of Nation's Infected Population
0	100.00%	0	0.00%	11.48%
0	100.00%	0	0.00%	11.48%
3,107,386	100.00%	0	0.00%	11.48%
2,905,314	39.70%	4,412,234	3.72%	4.56%
2,676,393	100.00%	0	0.00%	11.48%
1,088,080	12.31%	7,749,898	6.53%	1.41%
1,000,468	10.55%	8,483,314	7.15%	1.21%
958,075	27.71%	2,499,701	2.11%	3.18%
926,987	28.45%	2,330,815	1.96%	3.27%
719,263	28.70%	1,786,586	1.51%	3.29%
568,062	20.43%	2,212,698	1.86%	2.34%
558,171	19.39%	2,320,254	1.95%	2.23%
552,518	30.81%	1,240,617	1.05%	3.54%
512,952	12.43%	3,613,554	3.04%	1.43%
477,625	27.24%	1,275,842	1.07%	3.13%
426,753	4.36%	9,355,625	7.88%	.50%
414,035	5.00%	7,863,052	6.62%	.57%
286,857	6.77%	3,947,468	3.33%	.78%
281,205	5.39%	4,931,622	4.15%	.62%
245,878	11.52%	1,887,604	1.59%	1.32%
243,052	6.95%	3,254,699	2.74%	.80%
206,311	4.13%	4,793,135	4.04%	.47%
179,462	8.13%	2,026,745	1.71%	.93%
165,332	28.94%	406,036	.34%	3.32%
161,092	5.88%	2,577,502	2.17%	.68%
142,722	3.36%	4,108,862	3.46%	.39%
141,309	3.23%	4,228,038	3.56%	.37%
139,896	5.20%	2,552,582	2.15%	.60%
110,221	20.48%	428,056	.36%	2.35%
105,982	2.91%	3,535,776	2.98%	.33%
94,677	2.76%	3,340,343	2.81%	.32%
91,851	4.28%	2,053,872	1.73%	.49%
89,025	12.11%	646,340	.54%	1.39%
83,372	6.60%	1,179,322	.99%	.76%
74,894	6.66%	1,049,915	.88%	.76%
72,068	3.41%	2,042,919	1.72%	.39%
67,828	15.67%	365,125	.31%	1.80%
62,176	2.62%	2,310,545	1.95%	.30%
56,524	2.03%	2,722,815	2.29%	.23%
55,111	5.54%	938,809	.79%	.64%
39,567	4.79%	786,915	.66%	.55%
35,327	2.38%	1,450,454	1.22%	.27%
35,327	11.12%	282,480	.24%	1.28%
31,088	1.66%	1,845,233	1.55%	.19%
15,544	3.28%	458,933	.39%	.38%
11,305	1.23%	905,839	.76%	.14%
9,892	1.30%	753,266	.63%	.15%
9,892	2.22%	436,133	.37%	.25%
5,652	.83%	671,669	.57%	.10%
5,652	.88%	633,618	.53%	.10%
20,248,173		118,696,858	100%	100%

47.46%

1996 infect. 107,211,960

AIDS Projections by State
Assuming AIDS Distribution
Proportionate to a State's
Population.

STATE	1980 CENSUS STATE'S TOTAL POPULATION	CDC March '87 Diagnosed Cases by State (1986)	Estimated % Total Infect AIDS Populat
New York	17,558,072	10091	31.63%
California	23,667,565	7486	23.46%
Florida	9,746,324	2199	6.89%
Texas	14,229,288	2056	6.44%
New Jersey	7,364,823	1894	5.94%
Illinois	11,426,518	770	2.41%
Pennsylvania	11,863,895	708	2.22%
Massachuestts	5,737,037	678	2.12%
Georgia	5,463,105	656	2.06%
Maryland	4,216,975	509	1.60%
Washington	4,132,180	402	1.26%
Louisiana	4,206,312	395	1.24%
Conneticut	3,107,576	391	1.23%
Virginia	5,346,818	363	1.14%
Colorado	2,889,735	338	1.06%
Ohio	10,797,624	302	.95%
Michigan	9,262,078	293	.92%
Missouri	4,916,759	203	.64%
North Carolin	5,881,813	199	.62%
Arizona	2,718,425	174	.55%
Minnesota	4,075,970	172	.54%
Indiana	5,490,260	146	.46%
Oregon	2,633,149	127	.40%
Hawaii	964,691	117	.37%
South Carolin	3,121,833	114	.36%
Tennessee	4,591,120	101	.32%
Wisconsin	4,705,521	100	.31%
Oklahoma	3,025,290	99	.31%
Nevada	800,493	78	.24%
Alabama	3,893,888	75	.24%
Kentucky	3,660,257	67	.21%
Kansas	2,364,236	65	.20%
Rhode Island	947,154	63	.20%
Utah	1,461,037	59	.18%
New Mexico	1,302,981	53	.17%
Arkansas	2,286,435	51	.16%
Delaware	594,317	48	.15%
Mississippi	2,520,638	44	.14%
Iowa	2,913,808	40	.13%
Maine	1,125,027	39	.12%
New Hampshire	920,610	28	.09%
Nebraska	1,569,825	25	.08%
Alaska	401,851	25	.08%
West Virginia	1,950,279	22	.07%
Vermont	511,456	11	.03%
Idaho	944,038	8	.03%
Montana	786,690	7	.02%
Wyoming	469,557	7	.02%
South Dakota	690,768	4	.01%
North Dakota	652,717	4	.01%
	225,908,818	31906	100%

Percent of Nation's Pop. >
Now Infected this Year

Infected Total in 1997 63,120,489	Percent of State's Population Infected	Remaining Non-infected In State	Percent of Nation's Non-infected Population	State's Pop. Weighted Percent of Nation's Infected Population
0	100.00%	0	0.00%	8.06%
0	100.00%	0	0.00%	8.06%
0	100.00%	0	0.00%	8.06%
4,067,440	92.19%	344,795	.35%	7.43%
0	100.00%	0	0.00%	8.06%
1,523,311	19.66%	6,226,586	6.32%	1.59%
1,400,655	16.51%	7,082,659	7.19%	1.33%
1,341,305	53.66%	1,158,396	1.18%	4.33%
1,297,782	55.68%	1,033,033	1.05%	4.49%
1,006,968	56.36%	779,617	.79%	4.55%
795,287	35.94%	1,417,410	1.44%	2.90%
781,439	33.68%	1,538,815	1.56%	2.72%
773,526	62.35%	467,091	.47%	5.03%
718,133	19.87%	2,895,422	2.94%	1.60%
668,674	52.41%	607,168	.62%	4.23%
597,455	6.39%	8,758,170	8.90%	.51%
579,650	7.37%	7,283,403	7.40%	.59%
401,600	10.17%	3,545,868	3.60%	.82%
393,687	7.98%	4,537,935	4.61%	.64%
344,229	18.24%	1,543,375	1.57%	1.47%
340,272	10.45%	2,914,427	2.96%	.84%
288,836	6.03%	4,504,299	4.58%	.49%
251,247	12.40%	1,775,498	1.80%	1.00%
231,464	57.01%	174,571	.18%	4.60%
225,529	8.75%	2,351,973	2.39%	.71%
199,811	4.86%	3,909,051	3.97%	.39%
197,833	4.68%	4,030,205	4.09%	.38%
195,854	7.67%	2,356,727	2.39%	.62%
154,309	36.05%	273,747	.28%	2.91%
148,374	4.20%	3,387,401	3.44%	.34%
132,548	3.97%	3,207,795	3.26%	.32%
128,591	6.26%	1,925,281	1.96%	.50%
124,635	19.28%	521,705	.53%	1.56%
116,721	9.90%	1,062,601	1.08%	.80%
104,851	9.99%	945,064	.96%	.81%
100,895	4.94%	1,942,024	1.97%	.40%
94,960	26.01%	270,165	.27%	2.10%
87,046	3.77%	2,223,499	2.26%	.30%
79,133	2.91%	2,643,682	2.69%	.23%
77,155	8.22%	861,654	.88%	.66%
55,393	7.04%	731,522	.74%	.57%
49,458	3.41%	1,400,996	1.42%	.27%
49,458	17.51%	233,022	.24%	1.41%
43,523	2.36%	1,801,710	1.83%	.19%
21,762	4.74%	437,171	.44%	.38%
15,827	1.75%	890,013	.90%	.14%
13,848	1.84%	739,418	.75%	.15%
13,848	3.18%	422,285	.43%	.26%
7,913	1.18%	663,755	.67%	.10%
7,913	1.25%	625,704	.64%	.10%
20,250,151		98,446,707	100%	100%
		56.42%		
		1997 infect. 127,462,111		

AIDS PROJECTIONS Based on December of Year Numbers and on Present Growth Rates and 1980 Census Data Year – Legend	Total Number of AIDS Cases Diagnosed This Year Only	Cummulative Number Diagnosed AIDS Cases from 1941 to Year
yr 1941 ------->	0	0
yr 1942 :	0	0
yr 1943 :	0	0
yr 1944 D	0	0
yr 1945 I	0	0
yr 1946 S	0	0
yr 1947 E	0	0
yr 1948 A	0	0
yr 1949 S	0	0
yr 1950 E	0	0
yr 1951 :	0	0
yr 1952 N	0	0
yr 1953 O	0	0
yr 1954 T	0	1
yr 1955 :	0	1
yr 1956 Y	0	1
yr 1957 E	1	2
yr 1958 T	1	2
yr 1959 :	1	3
yr 1960 R	1	5
yr 1961 E	2	7
yr 1962 C	3	9
yr 1963 O	4	13
yr 1964 G	5	18
yr 1965 N	7	26
yr 1966 I	10	36
yr 1967 Z	14	51
yr 1968 E	20	71
yr 1969 D	28	99
yr 1970 :	40	139
yr 1971 T	56	195
yr 1972 I	78	273
yr 1973 L	109	382
yr 1974 L	153	535
yr 1975 :	214	748
yr 1976 N	299	1,048
yr 1977 O	419	1,467
yr 1978 W	587	2,054
yr 1979 :	821	2,875
yr 1980 :	1,150	4,025
yr 1981 ------->	1,610	5,635
yr 1982 Virus	2,254	7,889
yr 1983 Found	3,156	11,045
yr 1984	4,418	15,463
yr 1985	6,185	21,649
yr 1986	8,659	30,308

Remaining Number of U.S. Citizens Not Diagnosed with AIDS to Year (1980 Census)	Total Number of New Infected AIDS Cases Beginning This Year Only	Average Number of New Infected AIDS Cases Beginning Per Day This Year Only
226,545,805	0	0
226,545,805	0	0
226,545,805	0	0
226,545,805	0	0
226,545,805	0	0
226,545,805	1	0
226,545,805	1	0
226,545,805	1	0
226,545,805	2	0
226,545,805	2	0
226,545,805	3	0
226,545,805	5	0
226,545,805	7	0
226,545,804	9	0
226,545,804	13	0
226,545,804	18	0
226,545,803	25	0
226,545,803	35	0
226,545,802	49	0
226,545,800	69	0
226,545,798	96	0
226,545,796	135	0
226,545,792	189	1
226,545,787	264	1
226,545,779	370	1
226,545,769	517	1
226,545,754	724	2
226,545,734	1,014	3
226,545,706	1,420	4
226,545,666	1,988	5
226,545,610	2,783	8
226,545,532	3,896	11
226,545,423	5,455	15
226,545,270	7,637	21
226,545,057	10,692	29
226,544,757	14,969	41
226,544,338	20,956	57
226,543,751	29,338	80
226,542,930	41,074	113
226,541,780	57,503	158
226,540,170	80,504	221
226,537,916	112,706	309
226,534,760	157,788	432
226,530,342	220,904	605
226,524,156	309,265	847
226,515,497	432,972	1,186

AIDS PROJECTIONS
Based on December
of Year Numbers
and on Present
Growth Rates and
1980 Census Data

Year	Legend	Total Number of AIDS Cases Diagnosed This Year Only	Cummulative Number Diagnosed AIDS Cases from 1941 to Year
yr 1987		12,123	42,431
yr 1988		16,972	59,404
yr 1989		23,761	83,165
yr 1990		33,266	116,431
yr 1991		46,573	163,004
yr 1992		65,202	228,205
yr 1993		91,282	319,487
yr 1994		127,795	447,282
yr 1995		178,913	626,195
yr 1996		250,478	876,673
yr 1997	------->	350,669	1,227,343
yr 1998	:	490,937	1,718,280
yr 1999	:	687,312	2,405,592
yr 2000	US infect	962,237	3,367,829
yr 2001	:	1,347,131	4,714,960
yr 2002	:	1,885,984	6,600,944
yr 2003	------->	2,640,378	9,241,322
yr 2004		3,696,529	12,937,850
yr 2005		5,175,140	18,112,991
yr 2006		7,245,196	25,358,187
yr 2007		10,143,275	35,501,462
yr 2008		14,200,585	49,702,046
yr 2009		19,880,819	69,582,865
yr 2010		27,833,146	97,416,011
yr 2011	------->	38,966,404	136,382,415
yr 2012	:	54,552,966	190,935,382
yr 2013	US diagno	76,374,153	267,309,534
yr 2014	:	106,923,814	374,233,348
yr 2015	------->	149,693,339	523,926,687
yr 2016	:	209,570,675	733,497,362
yr 2017	US dead	293,398,945	1,026,896,307
yr 2018	:	410,758,523	1,437,654,829
yr 2019	------->	575,061,932	2,012,716,761
yr 2020		805,086,704	2,817,803,466
yr 2021		1,127,121,386	3,944,924,852
yr 2022	------->	1,577,969,941	5,522,894,793
yr 2023	:	2,209,157,917	7,732,052,710
yr 2024	World dia	3,092,821,084	10,824,873,794
yr 2025	:	4,329,949,518	15,154,823,312
yr 2026	------->	6,061,929,325	21,216,752,636
yr 2027	:	8,486,701,054	29,703,453,691
yr 2028	World dea	11,881,381,476	41,584,835,167
yr 2029	:	16,633,934,067	58,218,769,234
yr 2030	------->	23,287,507,693	81,506,276,927

Remaining Number of U.S. Citizens Not Diagnosed with AIDS to Year (1980 Census)	Total Number of New Infected AIDS Cases Beginning This Year Only	Average Number of New Infected AIDS Cases Beginning Per Day This Year Only
226,503,374	606,160	1,661
226,486,401	848,624	2,325
226,462,640	1,188,074	3,255
226,429,374	1,663,304	4,557
226,382,801	2,328,625	6,380
226,317,600	3,260,076	8,932
226,226,318	4,564,106	12,504
226,098,523	6,389,748	17,506
225,919,610	8,945,647	24,509
225,669,132	12,523,906	34,312
225,318,462	17,533,469	48,037
224,827,525	24,546,856	67,252
224,140,213	34,365,598	94,152
223,177,976	48,111,838	131,813
221,830,845	67,356,573	184,539
219,944,861	94,299,202	258,354
217,304,483	132,018,883	361,696
213,607,955	184,826,436	506,374
208,432,814	258,757,010	708,923
201,187,618	362,259,814	992,493
191,044,343	507,163,739	1,389,490
176,843,759	710,029,235	1,945,286
156,962,940	994,040,929	2,723,400
129,129,794	1,391,657,300	3,812,760
90,163,390	1,948,320,220	5,337,864
35,610,423	2,727,648,309	7,473,009
(40,763,729)	3,818,707,632	10,462,213
(147,687,543)	5,346,190,685	14,647,098
(297,380,882)	7,484,666,959	20,505,937
(506,951,557)	10,478,533,742	28,708,312
(800,350,502)	14,669,947,239	40,191,636
(1,211,109,024)	20,537,926,135	56,268,291
(1,786,170,956)	28,753,096,589	78,775,607
(2,591,257,661)	40,254,335,225	110,285,850
(3,718,379,047)	56,356,069,315	154,400,190
(5,296,348,988)	78,898,497,040	216,160,266
(7,505,506,905)	110,457,895,857	302,624,372
(10,598,327,989)	154,641,054,199	423,674,121
(14,928,277,507)	216,497,475,879	593,143,770
(20,990,206,831)	303,096,466,230	830,401,277
(29,476,907,886)	424,335,052,723	1,162,561,788
(41,358,289,362)	594,069,073,812	1,627,586,504
(57,992,223,429)	831,696,703,336	2,278,621,105
(81,279,731,122)	1,164,375,384,671	3,190,069,547

AIDS PROJECTIONS
Based on December
of Year Numbers
and on Present
Growth Rates and
1980 Census Data

Year	Legend	Cummulative Number New Infected AIDS Cases from 1941 to Year	Remaining Number of U.S. Citizens Not Infected with AIDS to Year (1980 Census)
yr 1941	------->	0	226,545,805
yr 1942	:	0	226,545,805
yr 1943	:	1	226,545,804
yr 1944	D	1	226,545,804
yr 1945	I	1	226,545,804
yr 1946	S	2	226,545,803
yr 1947	E	3	226,545,802
yr 1948	A	4	226,545,801
yr 1949	S	6	226,545,799
yr 1950	E	8	226,545,797
yr 1951	:	11	226,545,794
yr 1952	N	16	226,545,789
yr 1953	O	23	226,545,782
yr 1954	T	32	226,545,773
yr 1955	:	44	226,545,761
yr 1956	Y	62	226,545,743
yr 1957	E	87	226,545,718
yr 1958	T	122	226,545,683
yr 1959	:	172	226,545,633
yr 1960	R	240	226,545,565
yr 1961	E	336	226,545,469
yr 1962	C	471	226,545,334
yr 1963	O	660	226,545,145
yr 1964	G	924	226,544,881
yr 1965	N	1,293	226,544,512
yr 1966	I	1,811	226,543,994
yr 1967	Z	2,535	226,543,270
yr 1968	E	3,550	226,542,255
yr 1969	D	4,970	226,540,835
yr 1970	:	6,958	226,538,847
yr 1971	T	9,741	226,536,064
yr 1972	I	13,637	226,532,168
yr 1973	L	19,092	226,526,713
yr 1974	L	26,729	226,519,076
yr 1975	:	37,421	226,508,384
yr 1976	N	52,390	226,493,415
yr 1977	O	73,345	226,472,460
yr 1978	W	102,684	226,443,121
yr 1979	:	143,757	226,402,048
yr 1980	:	201,261	226,344,544
yr 1981	------->	281,765	226,264,040
yr 1982	Virus	394,471	226,151,334
yr 1983	Found	552,259	225,993,546
yr 1984		773,163	225,772,642
yr 1985		1,082,429	225,463,376
yr 1986		1,515,400	225,030,405

Number of Deaths Per Year This Year Only	Average Number of Deaths Per Day This Year Only	Average Annual Life Insurance Disbursals This Year Only @ $25,000 Per Case
0	0	$37
0	0	$52
0	0	$73
0	0	$103
0	0	$144
0	0	$201
0	0	$281
0	0	$394
0	0	$552
0	0	$772
0	0	$1,081
0	0	$1,514
0	0	$2,119
0	0	$2,967
0	0	$4,153
0	0	$5,814
0	0	$8,140
0	0	$11,396
1	0	$15,955
1	0	$22,336
1	0	$31,271
2	0	$43,779
2	0	$61,291
3	0	$85,808
5	0	$120,131
7	0	$168,183
9	0	$235,456
13	0	$329,639
18	0	$461,494
26	0	$646,092
36	0	$904,529
51	0	$1,266,340
71	0	$1,772,876
99	0	$2,482,026
139	0	$3,474,837
195	1	$4,864,772
272	1	$6,810,680
381	1	$9,534,952
534	1	$13,348,933
748	2	$18,688,506
1,047	3	$26,163,909
1,465	4	$36,629,472
2,051	6	$51,281,261
2,872	8	$71,793,766
4,020	11	$100,511,272
5,629	15	$140,715,781

AIDS PROJECTIONS
Based on December
of Year Numbers
and on Present
Growth Rates and
1980 Census Data

Year - Legend		Cummulative Number New Infected AIDS Cases from 1941 to Year	Remaining Number of U.S. Citizens Not Infected with AIDS to Year (1980 Census)
yr 1987		2,121,561	224,424,244
yr 1988		2,970,185	223,575,620
yr 1989		4,158,259	222,387,546
yr 1990		5,821,563	220,724,242
yr 1991		8,150,188	218,395,617
yr 1992		11,410,264	215,135,541
yr 1993		15,974,370	210,571,435
yr 1994		22,364,118	204,181,687
yr 1995		31,309,765	195,236,040
yr 1996		43,833,671	182,712,134
yr 1997	------->	61,367,140	165,178,665
yr 1998	:	85,913,996	140,631,809
yr 1999	:	120,279,594	106,266,211
yr 2000	US infect	168,391,432	58,154,373
yr 2001	:	235,748,004	(9,202,199)
yr 2002	:	330,047,206	(103,501,401)
yr 2003	------->	462,066,089	(235,520,284)
yr 2004		646,892,524	(420,346,719)
yr 2005		905,649,534	(679,103,729)
yr 2006		1,267,909,348	(1,041,363,543)
yr 2007		1,775,073,087	(1,548,527,282)
yr 2008		2,485,102,322	(2,258,556,517)
yr 2009		3,479,143,250	(3,252,597,445)
yr 2010		4,870,800,551	(4,644,254,746)
yr 2011	------->	6,819,120,771	(6,592,574,966)
yr 2012	:	9,546,769,080	(9,320,223,275)
yr 2013	US diagno	13,365,476,712	(13,138,930,907)
yr 2014	:	18,711,667,397	(18,485,121,592)
yr 2015	------->	26,196,334,356	(25,969,788,551)
yr 2016	:	36,674,868,098	(36,448,322,293)
yr 2017	US dead	51,344,815,337	(51,118,269,532)
yr 2018	:	71,882,741,472	(71,656,195,667)
yr 2019	------->	100,635,838,061	(100,409,292,256)
yr 2020		140,890,173,286	(140,663,627,481)
yr 2021		197,246,242,601	(197,019,696,796)
yr 2022	------->	276,144,739,641	(275,918,193,836)
yr 2023	:	386,602,635,498	(386,376,089,693)
yr 2024	World dia	541,243,689,697	(541,017,143,892)
yr 2025	:	757,741,165,576	(757,514,619,771)
yr 2026	------->	1,060,837,631,806	(1,060,611,086,001)
yr 2027	:	1,485,172,684,529	(1,484,946,138,724)
yr 2028	World dea	2,079,241,758,341	(2,079,015,212,536)
yr 2029	:	2,910,938,461,677	(2,910,711,915,872)
yr 2030	------->	4,075,313,846,348	(4,075,087,300,543)

Number of Deaths Per Year This Year Only	Average Number of Deaths Per Day This Year Only	Average Annual Life Insurance Disbursals This Year Only @ $25,000 Per Case
7,880	22	$197,002,094
11,032	30	$275,802,932
15,445	42	$386,124,104
21,623	59	$540,573,746
30,272	83	$756,803,244
42,381	116	$1,059,524,542
59,333	163	$1,483,334,359
83,067	228	$2,076,668,103
116,293	319	$2,907,335,344
162,811	446	$4,070,269,481
227,935	624	$5,698,377,274
319,109	874	$7,977,728,184
446,753	1,224	$11,168,819,457
625,454	1,714	$15,636,347,240
875,635	2,399	$21,890,886,136
1,225,890	3,359	$30,647,240,591
1,716,245	4,702	$42,906,136,827
2,402,744	6,583	$60,068,591,558
3,363,841	9,216	$84,096,028,181
4,709,378	12,902	$117,734,439,453
6,593,129	18,063	$164,828,215,234
9,230,380	25,289	$230,759,501,327
12,922,532	35,404	$323,063,301,858
18,091,545	49,566	$452,288,622,602
25,328,163	69,392	$633,204,071,643
35,459,428	97,149	$886,485,700,300
49,643,199	136,009	$1,241,079,980,420
69,500,479	190,412	$1,737,511,972,587
97,300,670	266,577	$2,432,516,761,622
136,220,939	373,208	$3,405,523,466,271
190,709,314	522,491	$4,767,732,852,780
266,993,040	731,488	$6,674,825,993,892
373,790,256	1,024,083	$9,344,756,391,448
523,306,358	1,433,716	$13,082,658,948,028
732,628,901	2,007,202	$18,315,722,527,239
1,025,680,462	2,810,083	$25,642,011,538,134
1,435,952,646	3,934,117	$35,898,816,153,388
2,010,333,705	5,507,764	$50,258,342,614,743
2,814,467,186	7,710,869	$70,361,679,660,640
3,940,254,061	10,795,217	$98,506,351,524,896
5,516,355,685	15,113,303	$137,908,892,134,855
7,722,897,960	21,158,625	$193,072,448,988,797
10,812,057,143	29,622,074	$270,301,428,584,316
15,136,880,001	41,470,904	$378,422,000,018,042

AIDS PROJECTIONS
Based on December
of Year Numbers
and on Present
Growth Rates and
1980 Census Data

Year	– Legend	Average Daily Life Insurance Disbursals This Year Only @ $25,000 Per Case	Cummulative Number Deaths of AIDS Cases from 1941 to Year
yr 1941	------->	$0	0
yr 1942	:	$0	0
yr 1943	:	$0	0
yr 1944	D	$0	0
yr 1945	I	$0	0
yr 1946	S	$1	0
yr 1947	E	$1	0
yr 1948	A	$1	0
yr 1949	S	$2	0
yr 1950	E	$2	0
yr 1951	:	$3	0
yr 1952	N	$4	0
yr 1953	O	$6	0
yr 1954	T	$8	0
yr 1955	:	$11	1
yr 1956	Y	$16	1
yr 1957	E	$22	1
yr 1958	T	$31	2
yr 1959	:	$44	2
yr 1960	R	$61	3
yr 1961	E	$86	4
yr 1962	C	$120	6
yr 1963	O	$168	9
yr 1964	G	$235	12
yr 1965	N	$329	17
yr 1966	I	$461	24
yr 1967	Z	$645	33
yr 1968	E	$903	46
yr 1969	D	$1,264	65
yr 1970	:	$1,770	90
yr 1971	T	$2,478	127
yr 1972	I	$3,469	177
yr 1973	L	$4,857	248
yr 1974	L	$6,800	347
yr 1975	:	$9,520	486
yr 1976	N	$13,328	681
yr 1977	O	$18,659	953
yr 1978	W	$26,123	1,335
yr 1979	:	$36,572	1,869
yr 1980	:	$51,201	2,616
yr 1981	------->	$71,682	3,663
yr 1982	Virus	$100,355	5,128
yr 1983	Found	$140,497	7,179
yr 1984		$196,695	10,051
yr 1985		$275,373	14,072
yr 1986		$385,523	19,700

Cummulative Life Insurance Disbursals From 1941 to Year @ $25,000 Per Case	Remaining Number of U.S. Citizens Not Dead from AIDS to Year (1980 Census)	Remaining Living AIDS Cases This Year Only
$37	226,545,805	0
$90	226,545,805	0
$163	226,545,805	0
$266	226,545,805	0
$409	226,545,805	0
$610	226,545,805	0
$892	226,545,805	0
$1,286	226,545,805	0
$1,837	226,545,805	0
$2,609	226,545,805	0
$3,690	226,545,805	0
$5,204	226,545,805	0
$7,323	226,545,805	0
$10,289	226,545,805	1
$14,442	226,545,804	1
$20,257	226,545,804	1
$28,397	226,545,804	1
$39,793	226,545,803	2
$55,748	226,545,803	3
$78,084	226,545,802	4
$109,355	226,545,801	5
$153,135	226,545,799	8
$214,426	226,545,796	11
$300,233	226,545,793	15
$420,364	226,545,788	21
$588,547	226,545,781	29
$824,003	226,545,772	41
$1,153,642	226,545,759	58
$1,615,136	226,545,740	81
$2,261,228	226,545,715	113
$3,165,756	226,545,678	159
$4,432,096	226,545,628	222
$6,204,972	226,545,557	311
$8,686,999	226,545,458	435
$12,161,835	226,545,319	609
$17,026,607	226,545,124	853
$23,837,287	226,544,852	1,194
$33,372,239	226,544,470	1,672
$46,721,172	226,543,936	2,341
$65,409,679	226,543,189	3,278
$91,573,588	226,542,142	4,589
$128,203,060	226,540,677	6,424
$179,484,322	226,538,626	8,994
$251,278,088	226,535,754	12,592
$351,789,360	226,531,733	17,628
$492,505,142	226,526,105	24,679

AIDS PROJECTIONS
Based on December
of Year Numbers
and on Present
Growth Rates and
1980 Census Data

Year	Legend	Average Daily Life Insurance Disbursals This Year Only @ $25,000 Per Case	Cummulative Number Deaths of AIDS Cases from 1941 to Year
yr 1987		$539,732	27,580
yr 1988		$755,624	38,612
yr 1989		$1,057,874	54,057
yr 1990		$1,481,024	75,680
yr 1991		$2,073,434	105,952
yr 1992		$2,902,807	148,333
yr 1993		$4,063,930	207,667
yr 1994		$5,689,502	290,734
yr 1995		$7,965,302	407,027
yr 1996		$11,151,423	569,838
yr 1997	------->	$15,611,993	797,773
yr 1998	:	$21,856,790	1,116,882
yr 1999	:	$30,599,505	1,563,635
yr 2000	US infect	$42,839,308	2,189,089
yr 2001	:	$59,975,031	3,064,724
yr 2002	:	$83,965,043	4,290,614
yr 2003	------->	$117,551,060	6,006,859
yr 2004		$164,571,484	8,409,603
yr 2005		$230,400,077	11,773,444
yr 2006		$322,560,108	16,482,822
yr 2007		$451,584,151	23,075,950
yr 2008		$632,217,812	32,306,330
yr 2009		$885,104,937	45,228,862
yr 2010		$1,239,146,911	63,320,407
yr 2011	------->	$1,734,805,676	88,648,570
yr 2012	:	$2,428,727,946	124,107,998
yr 2013	US diagno	$3,400,219,124	173,751,197
yr 2014	:	$4,760,306,774	243,251,676
yr 2015	------->	$6,664,429,484	340,552,347
yr 2016	:	$9,330,201,277	476,773,285
yr 2017	US dead	$13,062,281,788	667,482,599
yr 2018	:	$18,287,194,504	934,475,639
yr 2019	------->	$25,602,072,305	1,308,265,895
yr 2020		$35,842,901,227	1,831,572,253
yr 2021		$50,180,061,718	2,564,201,154
yr 2022	------->	$70,252,086,406	3,589,881,615
yr 2023	:	$98,352,920,968	5,025,834,261
yr 2024	World dia	$137,694,089,355	7,036,167,966
yr 2025	:	$192,771,725,098	9,850,635,152
yr 2026	------->	$269,880,415,137	13,790,889,213
yr 2027	:	$377,832,581,191	19,307,244,899
yr 2028	World dea	$528,965,613,668	27,030,142,858
yr 2029	:	$740,551,859,135	37,842,200,002
yr 2030	------->	$1,036,772,602,789	52,979,080,003

Cummulative Life Insurance Disbursals From 1941 to Year @ $25,000 Per Case	Remaining Number of U.S. Citizens Not Dead from AIDS to Year (1980 Census)	Remaining Living AIDS Cases This Year Only
$689,507,236	226,518,225	34,551
$965,310,167	226,507,193	48,372
$1,351,434,272	226,491,748	67,720
$1,892,008,018	226,470,125	94,808
$2,648,811,262	226,439,853	132,732
$3,708,335,804	226,397,472	185,824
$5,191,670,164	226,338,138	260,154
$7,268,338,266	226,255,071	364,216
$10,175,673,610	226,138,778	509,902
$14,245,943,092	225,975,967	713,863
$19,944,320,366	225,748,032	999,408
$27,922,048,550	225,428,923	1,399,171
$39,090,868,007	224,982,170	1,958,839
$54,727,215,247	224,356,716	2,742,375
$76,618,101,383	223,481,081	3,839,325
$107,265,341,974	222,255,191	5,375,054
$150,171,478,800	220,538,946	7,525,076
$210,240,070,358	218,136,202	10,535,107
$294,336,098,539	214,772,361	14,749,150
$412,070,537,991	210,062,983	20,648,809
$576,898,753,225	203,469,855	28,908,333
$807,658,254,553	194,239,475	40,471,666
$1,130,721,556,411	181,316,943	56,660,333
$1,583,010,179,013	163,225,398	79,324,466
$2,216,214,250,656	137,897,235	111,054,253
$3,102,699,950,955	102,437,807	155,475,954
$4,343,779,931,375	52,794,608	217,666,335
$6,081,291,903,962	(16,705,871)	304,732,869
$8,513,808,665,585	(114,006,542)	426,626,017
$11,919,332,131,856	(250,227,480)	597,276,423
$16,687,064,984,636	(440,936,794)	836,186,993
$23,361,890,978,527	(707,929,834)	1,170,661,790
$32,706,647,369,976	(1,081,720,090)	1,638,926,506
$45,789,306,318,003	(1,605,026,448)	2,294,497,108
$64,105,028,845,242	(2,337,655,349)	3,212,295,951
$89,747,040,383,376	(3,363,335,810)	4,497,214,331
$125,645,856,536,764	(4,799,288,456)	6,296,100,064
$175,904,199,151,508	(6,809,622,161)	8,814,540,089
$246,265,878,812,148	(9,624,089,347)	12,340,356,125
$344,772,230,337,044	(13,564,343,408)	17,276,498,575
$482,681,122,471,899	(19,080,699,094)	24,187,098,005
$675,753,571,460,696	(26,803,597,053)	33,861,937,207
$946,055,000,045,012	(37,615,654,197)	47,406,712,090
$1,324,477,000,063,055	(52,752,534,198)	66,369,396,926

AIDS PROJECTIONS
Based on December
of Year Numbers
and on Present
Growth Rates and
1980 Census Data

Year	Legend	Cost of Medical Treatment for Living AIDS Patients This Year Only @ $36,750 per Case	Annual Federal Budget Required for AID Programming This Year Only to Keep 1987 Levls
yr 1941	------->	$30	$13
yr 1942	:	$126	$54
yr 1943	:	$261	$111
yr 1944	D	$450	$192
yr 1945	I	$714	$305
yr 1946	S	$1,084	$463
yr 1947	E	$1,603	$684
yr 1948	A	$2,328	$993
yr 1949	S	$3,344	$1,427
yr 1950	E	$4,766	$2,034
yr 1951	:	$6,757	$2,883
yr 1952	N	$9,544	$4,072
yr 1953	O	$13,446	$5,737
yr 1954	T	$18,909	$8,068
yr 1955	:	$26,557	$11,332
yr 1956	Y	$37,264	$15,901
yr 1957	E	$52,255	$22,297
yr 1958	T	$73,241	$31,252
yr 1959	:	$102,622	$43,789
yr 1960	R	$143,756	$61,341
yr 1961	E	$201,342	$85,913
yr 1962	C	$281,964	$120,314
yr 1963	O	$394,834	$168,476
yr 1964	G	$552,852	$235,902
yr 1965	N	$774,077	$330,299
yr 1966	I	$1,083,793	$462,454
yr 1967	Z	$1,517,394	$647,472
yr 1968	E	$2,124,437	$906,497
yr 1969	D	$2,974,296	$1,269,132
yr 1970	:	$4,164,099	$1,776,821
yr 1971	T	$5,829,823	$2,487,585
yr 1972	I	$8,161,837	$3,482,656
yr 1973	L	$11,426,656	$4,875,754
yr 1974	L	$15,997,403	$6,826,092
yr 1975	:	$22,396,448	$9,556,565
yr 1976	N	$31,355,112	$13,379,226
yr 1977	O	$43,897,242	$18,730,953
yr 1978	W	$61,456,223	$26,223,370
yr 1979	:	$86,038,797	$36,712,755
yr 1980	:	$120,454,400	$51,397,893
yr 1981	------->	$168,636,245	$71,957,086
yr 1982	Virus	$236,090,827	$100,739,956
yr 1983	Found	$330,527,242	$141,035,974
yr 1984		$462,738,224	$197,450,400
yr 1985		$647,833,598	$276,430,596
yr 1986		$906,967,122	$387,002,871

Annual Loss of Productivity in Dollars Resulting From AIDS	Total Economic Impact (Cost) of AIDS From All Sources In This Projection Sheet This Year Only
$2	$81
$8	$240
$16	$461
$27	$771
$43	$1,206
$66	$1,814
$97	$2,665
$141	$3,857
$203	$5,525
$289	$7,860
$409	$11,130
$578	$15,708
$815	$22,117
$1,146	$31,090
$1,609	$43,651
$2,258	$61,238
$3,167	$85,859
$4,438	$120,328
$6,219	$168,585
$8,712	$236,144
$12,201	$330,728
$17,087	$463,144
$23,927	$648,528
$33,503	$908,064
$46,909	$1,271,416
$65,678	$1,780,108
$91,954	$2,492,277
$128,741	$3,489,313
$180,242	$4,885,165
$252,344	$6,839,356
$353,287	$9,575,224
$494,607	$13,405,440
$692,455	$18,767,741
$969,443	$26,274,963
$1,357,225	$36,785,075
$1,900,120	$51,499,230
$2,660,173	$72,099,048
$3,724,247	$100,938,793
$5,213,951	$141,314,436
$7,299,537	$197,840,336
$10,219,356	$276,976,596
$14,307,104	$387,767,360
$20,029,951	$542,874,429
$28,041,936	$760,024,326
$39,258,716	$1,064,034,183
$54,962,208	$1,489,647,981

AIDS PROJECTIONS
Based on December
of Year Numbers
and on Present
Growth Rates and
1980 Census Data

Year	Legend	Cost of Medical Treatment for Living AIDS Patients This Year Only @ $36,750 per Case	Annual Federal Budget Required for AID Programming This Year Only to Keep 1987 Levls
yr 1987		$1,269,754,055	$541,804,055
yr 1988		$1,777,655,761	$758,525,713
yr 1989		$2,488,718,150	$1,061,936,035
yr 1990		$3,484,205,495	$1,486,710,485
yr 1991		$4,877,887,777	$2,081,394,715
yr 1992		$6,829,042,973	$2,913,952,637
yr 1993		$9,560,660,247	$4,079,533,727
yr 1994		$13,384,924,430	$5,711,347,254
yr 1995		$18,738,894,286	$7,995,886,192
yr 1996		$26,234,452,085	$11,194,240,705
yr 1997	------->	$36,728,233,004	$15,671,937,023
yr 1998	:	$51,419,526,290	$21,940,711,868
yr 1999	:	$71,987,336,890	$30,716,996,651
yr 2000	US infect	$100,782,271,731	$43,003,795,348
yr 2001	:	$141,095,180,508	$60,205,313,523
yr 2002	:	$197,533,252,795	$84,287,438,968
yr 2003	------->	$276,546,553,998	$118,002,414,591
yr 2004		$387,165,175,682	$165,203,380,463
yr 2005		$542,031,246,039	$231,284,732,685
yr 2006		$758,843,744,539	$323,798,625,795
yr 2007		$1,062,381,242,439	$453,318,076,149
yr 2008		$1,487,333,739,499	$634,645,306,644
yr 2009		$2,082,267,235,383	$888,503,429,338
yr 2010		$2,915,174,129,620	$1,243,904,801,109
yr 2011	------->	$4,081,243,781,553	$1,741,466,721,589
yr 2012	:	$5,713,741,294,259	$2,438,053,410,260
yr 2013	US diagno	$7,999,237,812,047	$3,413,274,774,400
yr 2014	:	$11,198,932,936,950	$4,778,584,684,197
yr 2015	------->	$15,678,506,111,814	$6,690,018,557,911
yr 2016	:	$21,949,908,556,625	$9,366,025,981,112
yr 2017	US dead	$30,729,871,979,359	$13,112,436,373,593
yr 2018	:	$43,021,820,771,187	$18,357,410,923,066
yr 2019	------->	$60,230,549,079,747	$25,700,375,292,328
yr 2020		$84,322,768,711,730	$35,980,525,409,295
yr 2021		$118,051,876,196,507	$50,372,735,573,049
yr 2022	------->	$165,272,626,675,194	$70,521,829,802,305
yr 2023	:	$231,381,677,345,356	$98,730,561,723,263
yr 2024	World dia	$323,934,348,283,583	$138,222,786,412,605
yr 2025	:	$453,508,087,597,101	$193,511,900,977,683
yr 2026	------->	$634,911,322,636,025	$270,916,661,368,792
yr 2027	:	$888,875,851,690,520	$379,283,325,916,345
yr 2028	World dea	$1,244,426,192,366,812	$530,996,656,282,919
yr 2029	:	$1,742,196,669,313,622	$743,395,318,796,122
yr 2030	------->	$2,439,075,337,039,156	$1,040,753,446,314,608

Annual Loss of Productivity in Dollars Resulting From AIDS	Total Economic Impact (Cost) of AIDS From All Sources In This Projection Sheet This Year Only
$76,947,096	$2,085,507,300
$107,725,939	$2,919,710,345
$150,816,320	$4,087,594,609
$211,142,853	$5,722,632,579
$295,599,999	$8,011,685,736
$413,840,004	$11,216,360,156
$579,376,011	$15,702,904,344
$811,126,420	$21,984,066,207
$1,135,576,994	$30,777,692,816
$1,589,807,796	$43,088,770,068
$2,225,730,920	$60,324,278,221
$3,116,023,293	$84,453,989,634
$4,362,432,616	$118,235,585,614
$6,107,405,667	$165,529,819,985
$8,550,367,939	$231,741,748,105
$11,970,515,119	$324,438,447,473
$16,758,721,172	$454,213,826,588
$23,462,209,646	$635,899,357,349
$32,847,093,510	$890,259,100,414
$45,985,930,919	$1,246,362,740,705
$64,380,303,292	$1,744,907,837,113
$90,132,424,614	$2,442,870,972,084
$126,185,394,464	$3,420,019,361,043
$176,659,552,255	$4,788,027,105,586
$247,323,373,162	$6,703,237,947,946
$346,252,722,432	$9,384,533,127,251
$484,753,811,410	$13,138,346,378,277
$678,655,335,979	$18,393,684,929,713
$950,117,470,376	$25,751,158,901,724
$1,330,164,458,531	$36,051,622,462,539
$1,862,230,241,949	$50,472,271,447,681
$2,607,122,338,734	$70,661,180,026,879
$3,649,971,274,233	$98,925,652,037,756
$5,109,959,783,931	$138,495,912,852,984
$7,153,943,697,508	$193,894,277,994,303
$10,015,521,176,517	$271,451,989,192,150
$14,021,729,647,129	$380,032,784,869,136
$19,630,421,505,985	$532,045,898,816,916
$27,482,590,108,384	$744,864,258,343,808
$38,475,626,151,743	$1,042,809,961,681,457
$53,865,876,612,446	$1,459,933,946,354,166
$75,412,227,257,429	$2,043,907,524,895,958
$105,577,118,160,406	$2,861,470,534,854,466
$147,807,965,424,573	$4,006,058,748,796,378

AIDS PROJECTIONS
Based on December
of Year Numbers
and on Present
Growth Rates and
1980 Census Data

Year - Legend		Annual Percent of 1984 Gross National Product Lost by AIDS (All Sources) In 1972 Constant Dollars	Annual Medical Costs as a Percent of the 1987 Total U.S. Federal Budget
yr 1941	-------->	.0000%	.0000%
yr 1942	:	.0000%	.0000%
yr 1943	:	.0000%	.0000%
yr 1944	D	.0000%	.0000%
yr 1945	I	.0000%	.0000%
yr 1946	S	.0000%	.0000%
yr 1947	E	.0000%	.0000%
yr 1948	A	.0000%	.0000%
yr 1949	S	.0000%	.0000%
yr 1950	E	.0000%	.0000%
yr 1951	:	.0000%	.0000%
yr 1952	N	.0000%	.0000%
yr 1953	O	.0000%	.0000%
yr 1954	T	.0000%	.0000%
yr 1955	:	.0000%	.0000%
yr 1956	Y	.0000%	.0000%
yr 1957	E	.0000%	.0000%
yr 1958	T	.0000%	.0000%
yr 1959	:	.0000%	.0000%
yr 1960	R	.0000%	.0000%
yr 1961	E	.0000%	.0000%
yr 1962	C	.0000%	.0000%
yr 1963	O	.0000%	.0000%
yr 1964	G	.0001%	.0001%
yr 1965	N	.0001%	.0001%
yr 1966	I	.0001%	.0001%
yr 1967	Z	.0002%	.0002%
yr 1968	E	.0002%	.0002%
yr 1969	D	.0003%	.0003%
yr 1970	:	.0004%	.0004%
yr 1971	T	.0006%	.0006%
yr 1972	I	.0008%	.0008%
yr 1973	L	.0011%	.0011%
yr 1974	L	.0016%	.0016%
yr 1975	:	.0022%	.0022%
yr 1976	N	.0031%	.0031%
yr 1977	O	.0044%	.0044%
yr 1978	W	.0062%	.0061%
yr 1979	:	.0086%	.0086%
yr 1980	:	.0121%	.0120%
yr 1981	-------->	.0169%	.0169%
yr 1982	Virus	.0237%	.0236%
yr 1983	Found	.0331%	.0331%
yr 1984		.0464%	.0463%
yr 1985		.0649%	.0648%
yr 1986		.0909%	.0907%

Cummulative Number Remaining Alive AIDS Cases from 1941 to Year	Cummulative Cost Medical Treatment for AIDS Cases from 1941 to Year	Remaining Number of U.S. Citizens Not a Living AIDS Case to Year (1980 Census)
0	$30	226,545,805
0	$156	226,545,805
0	$416	226,545,805
0	$866	226,545,805
0	$1,580	226,545,805
0	$2,664	226,545,805
0	$4,267	226,545,805
0	$6,595	226,545,805
0	$9,939	226,545,805
0	$14,705	226,545,805
1	$21,461	226,545,804
1	$31,005	226,545,804
1	$44,451	226,545,804
2	$63,360	226,545,803
2	$89,917	226,545,803
3	$127,182	226,545,802
5	$179,437	226,545,800
7	$252,678	226,545,798
10	$355,300	226,545,795
14	$499,056	226,545,791
19	$700,398	226,545,786
27	$982,362	226,545,778
37	$1,377,196	226,545,768
53	$1,930,048	226,545,752
74	$2,704,125	226,545,731
103	$3,787,918	226,545,702
144	$5,305,312	226,545,661
202	$7,429,749	226,545,603
283	$10,404,045	226,545,522
396	$14,568,144	226,545,409
555	$20,397,967	226,545,250
777	$28,559,804	226,545,028
1,088	$39,986,460	226,544,717
1,523	$55,983,863	226,544,282
2,133	$78,380,311	226,543,672
2,986	$109,735,423	226,542,819
4,180	$153,632,665	226,541,625
5,853	$215,088,888	226,539,952
8,194	$301,127,685	226,537,611
11,472	$421,582,085	226,534,333
16,060	$590,218,330	226,529,745
22,485	$826,309,157	226,523,320
31,479	$1,156,836,399	226,514,326
44,070	$1,619,574,623	226,501,735
61,698	$2,267,408,221	226,484,107
86,378	$3,174,375,343	226,459,427

AIDS PROJECTIONS
Based on December
of Year Numbers
and on Present
Growth Rates and
1980 Census Data

Year - Legend	Annual Percent of 1984 Gross National Product Lost by AIDS (All Sources) In 1972 Constant Dollars	Annual Medical Costs as a Percent of the 1987 Total U.S. Federal Budget
yr 1987	.1272%	.1270%
yr 1988	.1781%	.1778%
yr 1989	.2494%	.2489%
yr 1990	.3492%	.3484%
yr 1991	.4888%	.4878%
yr 1992	.6843%	.6829%
yr 1993	.9581%	.9561%
yr 1994	1.3413%	1.3385%
yr 1995	1.8778%	1.8739%
yr 1996	2.6290%	2.6234%
yr 1997 -------->	3.6806%	3.6728%
yr 1998 :	5.1528%	5.1420%
yr 1999 :	7.2139%	7.1987%
yr 2000 US infect	10.0994%	10.0782%
yr 2001 :	14.1392%	14.1095%
yr 2002 :	19.7949%	19.7533%
yr 2003 -------->	27.7129%	27.6547%
yr 2004	38.7980%	38.7165%
yr 2005	54.3172%	54.2031%
yr 2006	76.0441%	75.8844%
yr 2007	106.4617%	106.2381%
yr 2008	149.0464%	148.7334%
yr 2009	208.6650%	208.2267%
yr 2010	292.1310%	291.5174%
yr 2011 ------->	408.9834%	408.1244%
yr 2012 :	572.5768%	571.3741%
yr 2013 US diagno	801.6075%	799.9238%
yr 2014 :	1122.2505%	1119.8933%
yr 2015 ------->	1571.1506%	1567.8506%
yr 2016 :	2199.6109%	2194.9909%
yr 2017 US dead	3079.4552%	3072.9872%
yr 2018 :	4311.2373%	4302.1821%
yr 2019 ------->	6035.7323%	6023.0549%
yr 2020	8450.0252%	8432.2769%
yr 2021	11830.0353%	11805.1876%
yr 2022 ------->	16562.0494%	16527.2627%
yr 2023 :	23186.8691%	23138.1677%
yr 2024 World dia	32461.6168%	32393.4348%
yr 2025 :	45446.2635%	45350.8088%
yr 2026 ------->	63624.7689%	63491.1323%
yr 2027 :	89074.6764%	88887.5852%
yr 2028 World dea	124704.5470%	124442.6192%
yr 2029 :	174586.3658%	174219.6669%
yr 2030 ------->	244420.9121%	243907.5337%

Cummulative Number Remaining Alive AIDS Cases from 1941 to Year	Cummulative Cost Medical Treatment for AIDS Cases from 1941 to Year	Remaining Number of U.S. Citizens Not a Living AIDS Case to Year (1980 Census)
120,929	$4,444,129,397	226,424,876
169,300	$6,221,785,159	226,376,505
237,020	$8,710,503,309	226,308,785
331,829	$12,194,708,804	226,213,976
464,560	$17,072,596,581	226,081,245
650,385	$23,901,639,554	225,895,420
910,539	$33,462,299,801	225,635,266
1,274,754	$46,847,224,231	225,271,051
1,784,656	$65,586,118,517	224,761,149
2,498,519	$91,820,570,602	224,047,286
3,497,927	$128,548,803,606	223,047,878
4,897,097	$179,968,329,895	221,648,708
6,855,937	$251,955,666,786	219,689,868
9,598,311	$352,737,938,516	216,947,494
13,437,636	$493,833,119,024	213,108,169
18,812,690	$691,366,371,819	207,733,115
26,337,767	$967,912,925,817	200,208,038
36,872,874	$1,355,078,101,499	189,672,931
51,622,023	$1,897,109,347,537	174,923,782
72,270,832	$2,655,953,092,076	154,274,973
101,179,166	$3,718,334,334,515	125,366,639
141,650,832	$5,205,668,074,014	84,894,973
198,311,165	$7,287,935,309,396	28,234,640
277,635,631	$10,203,109,439,017	(51,089,826)
388,689,884	$14,284,353,220,570	(162,144,079)
544,165,837	$19,998,094,514,828	(317,620,032)
761,832,172	$27,997,332,326,875	(535,286,367)
1,066,565,041	$39,196,265,263,825	(840,019,236)
1,493,191,058	$54,874,771,375,640	(1,266,645,253)
2,090,467,481	$76,824,679,932,264	(1,863,921,676)
2,926,654,474	$107,554,551,911,624	(2,700,108,669)
4,097,316,263	$150,576,372,682,811	(3,870,770,458)
5,736,242,769	$210,806,921,762,558	(5,509,696,964)
8,030,739,877	$295,129,690,474,288	(7,804,194,072)
11,243,035,828	$413,181,566,670,795	(11,016,490,023)
15,740,250,159	$578,454,193,345,989	(15,513,704,354)
22,036,350,223	$809,835,870,691,345	(21,809,804,418)
30,850,890,312	$1,133,770,218,974,928	(30,624,344,507)
43,191,246,437	$1,587,278,306,572,029	(42,964,700,632)
60,467,745,012	$2,222,189,629,208,054	(60,241,199,207)
84,654,843,018	$3,111,065,480,898,574	(84,428,297,213)
118,516,780,225	$4,355,491,673,265,386	(118,290,234,420)
165,923,492,315	$6,097,688,342,579,008	(165,696,946,510)
232,292,889,241	$8,536,763,679,618,164	(232,066,343,436)

AIDS PROJECTIONS
Based on December
of Year Numbers
and on Present
Growth Rates and
1980 Census Data

Year - Legend	Percent Alive to Diagnosed This Year	Percent Alive to Dead This Year	Percent Diagnosed to Alive this Year Only
yr 1941 -------->	35.00%	53.85%	285.71%
yr 1942 :	106.43%	163.74%	93.96%
yr 1943 :	157.45%	242.23%	63.51%
yr 1944 D	193.89%	298.30%	51.58%
yr 1945 I	219.92%	338.34%	45.47%
yr 1946 S	238.52%	366.95%	41.93%
yr 1947 E	251.80%	387.38%	39.71%
yr 1948 A	261.28%	401.98%	38.27%
yr 1949 S	268.06%	412.40%	37.31%
yr 1950 E	272.90%	419.85%	36.64%
yr 1951 :	276.36%	425.16%	36.19%
yr 1952 N	278.83%	428.96%	35.86%
yr 1953 O	280.59%	431.68%	35.64%
yr 1954 T	281.85%	433.62%	35.48%
yr 1955 :	282.75%	435.00%	35.37%
yr 1956 Y	283.39%	435.99%	35.29%
yr 1957 E	283.85%	436.70%	35.23%
yr 1958 T	284.18%	437.20%	35.19%
yr 1959 :	284.41%	437.56%	35.16%
yr 1960 R	284.58%	437.82%	35.14%
yr 1961 E	284.70%	438.00%	35.12%
yr 1962 C	284.79%	438.13%	35.11%
yr 1963 O	284.85%	438.23%	35.11%
yr 1964 G	284.89%	438.29%	35.10%
yr 1965 N	284.92%	438.34%	35.10%
yr 1966 I	284.94%	438.38%	35.09%
yr 1967 Z	284.96%	438.40%	35.09%
yr 1968 E	284.97%	438.42%	35.09%
yr 1969 D	284.98%	438.43%	35.09%
yr 1970 :	284.99%	438.44%	35.09%
yr 1971 T	284.99%	438.45%	35.09%
yr 1972 I	284.99%	438.45%	35.09%
yr 1973 L	284.99%	438.45%	35.09%
yr 1974 L	285.00%	438.46%	35.09%
yr 1975 :	285.00%	438.46%	35.09%
yr 1976 N	285.00%	438.46%	35.09%
yr 1977 O	285.00%	438.46%	35.09%
yr 1978 W	285.00%	438.46%	35.09%
yr 1979 :	285.00%	438.46%	35.09%
yr 1980 :	285.00%	438.46%	35.09%
yr 1981 -------->	285.00%	438.46%	35.09%
yr 1982 Virus	285.00%	438.46%	35.09%
yr 1983 Found	285.00%	438.46%	35.09%
yr 1984	285.00%	438.46%	35.09%
yr 1985	285.00%	438.46%	35.09%
yr 1986	285.00%	438.46%	35.09%

Percent Diagnosed to New Infected This Year	Percent Diagnosed to Dead This Year	Percent New Infected to Alive This Year	Percent New Infected to Dead This Year	Percent New Infected to Diagnosed This Year
2.00%	153.85%	14285.71%	7692.31%	5000.00%
2.00%	153.85%	4697.99%	7692.31%	5000.00%
2.00%	153.85%	3175.63%	7692.31%	5000.00%
2.00%	153.85%	2578.75%	7692.31%	5000.00%
2.00%	153.85%	2273.52%	7692.31%	5000.00%
2.00%	153.85%	2096.29%	7692.31%	5000.00%
2.00%	153.85%	1985.72%	7692.31%	5000.00%
2.00%	153.85%	1913.63%	7692.31%	5000.00%
2.00%	153.85%	1865.25%	7692.31%	5000.00%
2.00%	153.85%	1832.17%	7692.31%	5000.00%
2.00%	153.85%	1809.25%	7692.31%	5000.00%
2.00%	153.85%	1793.23%	7692.31%	5000.00%
2.00%	153.85%	1781.96%	7692.31%	5000.00%
2.00%	153.85%	1773.99%	7692.31%	5000.00%
2.00%	153.85%	1768.35%	7692.31%	5000.00%
2.00%	153.85%	1764.33%	7692.31%	5000.00%
2.00%	153.85%	1761.48%	7692.31%	5000.00%
2.00%	153.85%	1759.45%	7692.31%	5000.00%
2.00%	153.85%	1758.00%	7692.31%	5000.00%
2.00%	153.85%	1756.96%	7692.31%	5000.00%
2.00%	153.85%	1756.23%	7692.31%	5000.00%
2.00%	153.85%	1755.70%	7692.31%	5000.00%
2.00%	153.85%	1755.32%	7692.31%	5000.00%
2.00%	153.85%	1755.06%	7692.31%	5000.00%
2.00%	153.85%	1754.86%	7692.31%	5000.00%
2.00%	153.85%	1754.73%	7692.31%	5000.00%
2.00%	153.85%	1754.63%	7692.31%	5000.00%
2.00%	153.85%	1754.56%	7692.31%	5000.00%
2.00%	153.85%	1754.51%	7692.31%	5000.00%
2.00%	153.85%	1754.47%	7692.31%	5000.00%
2.00%	153.85%	1754.45%	7692.31%	5000.00%
2.00%	153.85%	1754.43%	7692.31%	5000.00%
2.00%	153.85%	1754.42%	7692.31%	5000.00%
2.00%	153.85%	1754.41%	7692.31%	5000.00%
2.00%	153.85%	1754.40%	7692.31%	5000.00%
2.00%	153.85%	1754.40%	7692.31%	5000.00%
2.00%	153.85%	1754.39%	7692.31%	5000.00%
2.00%	153.85%	1754.39%	7692.31%	5000.00%
2.00%	153.85%	1754.39%	7692.31%	5000.00%
2.00%	153.85%	1754.39%	7692.31%	5000.00%
2.00%	153.85%	1754.39%	7692.31%	5000.00%
2.00%	153.85%	1754.39%	7692.31%	5000.00%
2.00%	153.85%	1754.39%	7692.31%	5000.00%
2.00%	153.85%	1754.39%	7692.31%	5000.00%
2.00%	153.85%	1754.39%	7692.31%	5000.00%
2.00%	153.85%	1754.39%	7692.31%	5000.00%

AIDS PROJECTIONS
Based on December
of Year Numbers
and on Present
Growth Rates and
1980 Census Data

Year - Legend	Percent Alive to Diagnosed This Year	Percent Alive to Dead This Year	Percent Diagnosed to Alive this Year Only
yr 1987	285.00%	438.46%	35.09%
yr 1988	285.00%	438.46%	35.09%
yr 1989	285.00%	438.46%	35.09%
yr 1990	285.00%	438.46%	35.09%
yr 1991	285.00%	438.46%	35.09%
yr 1992	285.00%	438.46%	35.09%
yr 1993	285.00%	438.46%	35.09%
yr 1994	285.00%	438.46%	35.09%
yr 1995	285.00%	438.46%	35.09%
yr 1996	285.00%	438.46%	35.09%
yr 1997 ------->	285.00%	438.46%	35.09%
yr 1998 :	285.00%	438.46%	35.09%
yr 1999 :	285.00%	438.46%	35.09%
yr 2000 US infect	285.00%	438.46%	35.09%
yr 2001 :	285.00%	438.46%	35.09%
yr 2002 :	285.00%	438.46%	35.09%
yr 2003 ------->	285.00%	438.46%	35.09%
yr 2004	285.00%	438.46%	35.09%
yr 2005	285.00%	438.46%	35.09%
yr 2006	285.00%	438.46%	35.09%
yr 2007	285.00%	438.46%	35.09%
yr 2008	285.00%	438.46%	35.09%
yr 2009	285.00%	438.46%	35.09%
yr 2010	285.00%	438.46%	35.09%
yr 2011 ------->	285.00%	438.46%	35.09%
yr 2012 :	285.00%	438.46%	35.09%
yr 2013 US diagno	285.00%	438.46%	35.09%
yr 2014 :	285.00%	438.46%	35.09%
yr 2015 ------->	285.00%	438.46%	35.09%
yr 2016 :	285.00%	438.46%	35.09%
yr 2017 US dead	285.00%	438.46%	35.09%
yr 2018 :	285.00%	438.46%	35.09%
yr 2019 ------->	285.00%	438.46%	35.09%
yr 2020	285.00%	438.46%	35.09%
yr 2021	285.00%	438.46%	35.09%
yr 2022 ------->	285.00%	438.46%	35.09%
yr 2023 :	285.00%	438.46%	35.09%
yr 2024 World dia	285.00%	438.46%	35.09%
yr 2025 :	285.00%	438.46%	35.09%
yr 2026 ------->	285.00%	438.46%	35.09%
yr 2027 :	285.00%	438.46%	35.09%
yr 2028 World dea	285.00%	438.46%	35.09%
yr 2029 :	285.00%	438.46%	35.09%
yr 2030 ------->	285.00%	438.46%	35.09%

Percent Diagnosed to New Infected This Year	Percent Diagnosed to Dead This Year	Percent New Infected to Alive This Year	Percent New Infected to Dead This Year	Percent New Infected to Diagnosed This Year
2.00%	153.85%	1754.39%	7692.31%	5000.00%
2.00%	153.85%	1754.39%	7692.31%	5000.00%
2.00%	153.85%	1754.39%	7692.31%	5000.00%
2.00%	153.85%	1754.39%	7692.31%	5000.00%
2.00%	153.85%	1754.39%	7692.31%	5000.00%
2.00%	153.85%	1754.39%	7692.31%	5000.00%
2.00%	153.85%	1754.39%	7692.31%	5000.00%
2.00%	153.85%	1754.39%	7692.31%	5000.00%
2.00%	153.85%	1754.39%	7692.31%	5000.00%
2.00%	153.85%	1754.39%	7692.31%	5000.00%
2.00%	153.85%	1754.39%	7692.31%	5000.00%
2.00%	153.85%	1754.39%	7692.31%	5000.00%
2.00%	153.85%	1754.39%	7692.31%	5000.00%
2.00%	153.85%	1754.39%	7692.31%	5000.00%
2.00%	153.85%	1754.39%	7692.31%	5000.00%
2.00%	153.85%	1754.39%	7692.31%	5000.00%
2.00%	153.85%	1754.39%	7692.31%	5000.00%
2.00%	153.85%	1754.39%	7692.31%	5000.00%
2.00%	153.85%	1754.39%	7692.31%	5000.00%
2.00%	153.85%	1754.39%	7692.31%	5000.00%
2.00%	153.85%	1754.39%	7692.31%	5000.00%
2.00%	153.85%	1754.39%	7692.31%	5000.00%
2.00%	153.85%	1754.39%	7692.31%	5000.00%
2.00%	153.85%	1754.39%	7692.31%	5000.00%
2.00%	153.85%	1754.39%	7692.31%	5000.00%
2.00%	153.85%	1754.39%	7692.31%	5000.00%
2.00%	153.85%	1754.39%	7692.31%	5000.00%
2.00%	153.85%	1754.39%	7692.31%	5000.00%
2.00%	153.85%	1754.39%	7692.31%	5000.00%
2.00%	153.85%	1754.39%	7692.31%	5000.00%
2.00%	153.85%	1754.39%	7692.31%	5000.00%
2.00%	153.85%	1754.39%	7692.31%	5000.00%
2.00%	153.85%	1754.39%	7692.31%	5000.00%
2.00%	153.85%	1754.39%	7692.31%	5000.00%
2.00%	153.85%	1754.39%	7692.31%	5000.00%
2.00%	153.85%	1754.39%	7692.31%	5000.00%
2.00%	153.85%	1754.39%	7692.31%	5000.00%
2.00%	153.85%	1754.39%	7692.31%	5000.00%
2.00%	153.85%	1754.39%	7692.31%	5000.00%
2.00%	153.85%	1754.39%	7692.31%	5000.00%
2.00%	153.85%	1754.39%	7692.31%	5000.00%
2.00%	153.85%	1754.39%	7692.31%	5000.00%
2.00%	153.85%	1754.39%	7692.31%	5000.00%
2.00%	153.85%	1754.39%	7692.31%	5000.00%

AIDS PROJECTIONS
Based on December
of Year Numbers
and on Present
Growth Rates and
1980 Census Data

Year	Legend	Remaining Number of U.S. Citizens Not Living or Dead Case to Year (1980 Census)	Remaining Number of U.S. Citizens Not Diagnosed or Infected to Year (1980 Census)
yr 1987		226,397,296	224,381,813
yr 1988		226,337,892	223,516,216
yr 1989		226,254,727	222,304,381
yr 1990		226,138,296	220,607,811
yr 1991		225,975,292	218,232,613
yr 1992		225,747,087	214,907,336
yr 1993		225,427,599	210,251,948
yr 1994		224,980,317	203,734,405
yr 1995		224,354,122	194,609,845
yr 1996		223,477,448	181,835,461
yr 1997	------->	222,250,106	163,951,323
yr 1998	:	220,531,826	138,913,530
yr 1999	:	218,126,234	103,860,619
yr 2000	US infect	214,758,405	54,786,545
yr 2001	:	210,043,445	(13,917,159)
yr 2002	:	203,442,501	(110,102,345)
yr 2003	------->	194,201,179	(244,761,605)
yr 2004		181,263,329	(433,284,570)
yr 2005		163,150,338	(697,216,720)
yr 2006		137,792,151	(1,066,721,730)
yr 2007		102,290,689	(1,584,028,744)
yr 2008		52,588,643	(2,308,258,563)
yr 2009		(16,994,222)	(3,322,180,311)
yr 2010		(114,410,233)	(4,741,670,757)
yr 2011	------->	(250,792,649)	(6,728,957,382)
yr 2012	:	(441,728,030)	(9,511,158,656)
yr 2013	US diagno	(709,037,564)	(13,406,240,441)
yr 2014	:	(1,083,270,912)	(18,859,354,940)
yr 2015	------->	(1,607,197,599)	(26,493,715,238)
yr 2016	:	(2,340,694,961)	(37,181,819,655)
yr 2017	US dead	(3,367,591,268)	(52,145,165,839)
yr 2018	:	(4,805,246,098)	(73,093,850,497)
yr 2019	------->	(6,817,962,859)	(102,422,009,018)
yr 2020		(9,635,766,325)	(143,481,430,947)
yr 2021		(13,580,691,177)	(200,964,621,648)
yr 2022	------->	(19,103,585,969)	(281,441,088,629)
yr 2023	:	(26,835,638,679)	(394,108,142,403)
yr 2024	World dia	(37,660,512,473)	(551,842,017,686)
yr 2025	:	(52,815,335,785)	(772,669,443,082)
yr 2026	------->	(74,032,088,421)	(1,081,827,838,637)
yr 2027	:	(103,735,542,112)	(1,514,649,592,414)
yr 2028	World dea	(145,320,377,278)	(2,120,600,047,702)
yr 2029	:	(203,539,146,512)	(2,968,930,685,106)
yr 2030	------->	(285,045,423,439)	(4,156,593,577,470)

Remaining Number of U.S. Citizens Not Directly Impacted to Year (1980 Census)	Percent Dead to Alive this Year Only	Percent Dead to New Infected This Year	Percent Dead to Diagnosed This Year	Percent Alive to New Infected This Year
224,233,304	22.81%	1.30%	65.00%	5.70%
223,308,303	22.81%	1.30%	65.00%	5.70%
222,013,303	22.81%	1.30%	65.00%	5.70%
220,200,301	22.81%	1.30%	65.00%	5.70%
217,662,100	22.81%	1.30%	65.00%	5.70%
214,108,618	22.81%	1.30%	65.00%	5.70%
209,133,742	22.81%	1.30%	65.00%	5.70%
202,168,917	22.81%	1.30%	65.00%	5.70%
192,418,162	22.81%	1.30%	65.00%	5.70%
178,767,104	22.81%	1.30%	65.00%	5.70%
159,655,623	22.81%	1.30%	65.00%	5.70%
132,899,550	22.81%	1.30%	65.00%	5.70%
95,441,048	22.81%	1.30%	65.00%	5.70%
42,999,145	22.81%	1.30%	65.00%	5.70%
(30,419,519)	22.81%	1.30%	65.00%	5.70%
(133,205,649)	22.81%	1.30%	65.00%	5.70%
(277,106,231)	22.81%	1.30%	65.00%	5.70%
(478,567,046)	22.81%	1.30%	65.00%	5.70%
(760,612,187)	22.81%	1.30%	65.00%	5.70%
(1,155,475,384)	22.81%	1.30%	65.00%	5.70%
(1,708,283,859)	22.81%	1.30%	65.00%	5.70%
(2,482,215,725)	22.81%	1.30%	65.00%	5.70%
(3,565,720,338)	22.81%	1.30%	65.00%	5.70%
(5,082,626,795)	22.81%	1.30%	65.00%	5.70%
(7,206,295,835)	22.81%	1.30%	65.00%	5.70%
(10,179,432,492)	22.81%	1.30%	65.00%	5.70%
(14,341,823,811)	22.81%	1.30%	65.00%	5.70%
(20,169,171,657)	22.81%	1.30%	65.00%	5.70%
(28,327,458,642)	22.81%	1.30%	65.00%	5.70%
(39,749,060,421)	22.81%	1.30%	65.00%	5.70%
(55,739,302,912)	22.81%	1.30%	65.00%	5.70%
(78,125,642,399)	22.81%	1.30%	65.00%	5.70%
(109,466,517,682)	22.81%	1.30%	65.00%	5.70%
(153,343,743,076)	22.81%	1.30%	65.00%	5.70%
(214,771,858,629)	22.81%	1.30%	65.00%	5.70%
(300,771,220,403)	22.81%	1.30%	65.00%	5.70%
(421,170,326,887)	22.81%	1.30%	65.00%	5.70%
(589,729,075,964)	22.81%	1.30%	65.00%	5.70%
(825,711,324,672)	22.81%	1.30%	65.00%	5.70%
(1,156,086,472,863)	22.81%	1.30%	65.00%	5.70%
(1,618,611,680,331)	22.81%	1.30%	65.00%	5.70%
(2,266,146,970,786)	22.81%	1.30%	65.00%	5.70%
(3,172,696,377,422)	22.81%	1.30%	65.00%	5.70%
(4,441,865,546,714)	22.81%	1.30%	65.00%	5.70%

AIDS PROJECTIONS
Based on December
of Year Numbers
and on Present
Growth Rates and
1980 Census Data

Year	Legend	Remaining Number of U.S. Citizens Not Living or Dead Case to Year (1980 Census)	Remaining Number of U.S. Citizens Not Diagnosed or Infected to Year (1980 Census)
yr 1941	------->	226,545,805	226,545,805
yr 1942	:	226,545,805	226,545,805
yr 1943	:	226,545,805	226,545,804
yr 1944	D	226,545,805	226,545,804
yr 1945	I	226,545,805	226,545,804
yr 1946	S	226,545,805	226,545,803
yr 1947	E	226,545,805	226,545,802
yr 1948	A	226,545,805	226,545,801
yr 1949	S	226,545,805	226,545,799
yr 1950	E	226,545,804	226,545,797
yr 1951	:	226,545,804	226,545,793
yr 1952	N	226,545,804	226,545,789
yr 1953	O	226,545,803	226,545,782
yr 1954	T	226,545,803	226,545,773
yr 1955	:	226,545,802	226,545,760
yr 1956	Y	226,545,801	226,545,741
yr 1957	E	226,545,799	226,545,716
yr 1958	T	226,545,797	226,545,680
yr 1959	:	226,545,793	226,545,630
yr 1960	R	226,545,788	226,545,560
yr 1961	E	226,545,782	226,545,462
yr 1962	C	226,545,772	226,545,324
yr 1963	O	226,545,759	226,545,132
yr 1964	G	226,545,740	226,544,863
yr 1965	N	226,545,715	226,544,486
yr 1966	I	226,545,678	226,543,958
yr 1967	Z	226,545,628	226,543,219
yr 1968	E	226,545,557	226,542,184
yr 1969	D	226,545,457	226,540,736
yr 1970	:	226,545,318	226,538,708
yr 1971	T	226,545,123	226,535,869
yr 1972	I	226,544,851	226,531,895
yr 1973	L	226,544,469	226,526,331
yr 1974	L	226,543,934	226,518,541
yr 1975	:	226,543,186	226,507,636
yr 1976	N	226,542,138	226,492,368
yr 1977	O	226,540,671	226,470,993
yr 1978	W	226,538,617	226,441,068
yr 1979	:	226,535,742	226,399,172
yr 1980	:	226,531,717	226,340,519
yr 1981	------->	226,526,082	226,258,405
yr 1982	Virus	226,518,192	226,143,445
yr 1983	Found	226,507,147	225,982,500
yr 1984		226,491,684	225,757,178
yr 1985		226,470,035	225,441,728
yr 1986		226,439,727	225,000,097

Remaining Number of U.S. Citizens Not Directly Impacted to Year (1980 Census)	Percent Dead to Alive this Year Only	Percent Dead to New Infected This Year	Percent Dead to Diagnosed This Year	Percent Alive to New Infected This Year
226,545,805	185.71%	1.30%	65.00%	.70%
226,545,805	61.07%	1.30%	65.00%	2.13%
226,545,804	41.28%	1.30%	65.00%	3.15%
226,545,804	33.52%	1.30%	65.00%	3.88%
226,545,804	29.56%	1.30%	65.00%	4.40%
226,545,803	27.25%	1.30%	65.00%	4.77%
226,545,802	25.81%	1.30%	65.00%	5.04%
226,545,801	24.88%	1.30%	65.00%	5.23%
226,545,799	24.25%	1.30%	65.00%	5.36%
226,545,796	23.82%	1.30%	65.00%	5.46%
226,545,793	23.52%	1.30%	65.00%	5.53%
226,545,788	23.31%	1.30%	65.00%	5.58%
226,545,781	23.17%	1.30%	65.00%	5.61%
226,545,771	23.06%	1.30%	65.00%	5.64%
226,545,757	22.99%	1.30%	65.00%	5.66%
226,545,737	22.94%	1.30%	65.00%	5.67%
226,545,710	22.90%	1.30%	65.00%	5.68%
226,545,672	22.87%	1.30%	65.00%	5.68%
226,545,618	22.85%	1.30%	65.00%	5.69%
226,545,543	22.84%	1.30%	65.00%	5.69%
226,545,438	22.83%	1.30%	65.00%	5.69%
226,545,292	22.82%	1.30%	65.00%	5.70%
226,545,086	22.82%	1.30%	65.00%	5.70%
226,544,798	22.82%	1.30%	65.00%	5.70%
226,544,395	22.81%	1.30%	65.00%	5.70%
226,543,831	22.81%	1.30%	65.00%	5.70%
226,543,042	22.81%	1.30%	65.00%	5.70%
226,541,936	22.81%	1.30%	65.00%	5.70%
226,540,388	22.81%	1.30%	65.00%	5.70%
226,538,221	22.81%	1.30%	65.00%	5.70%
226,535,188	22.81%	1.30%	65.00%	5.70%
226,530,941	22.81%	1.30%	65.00%	5.70%
226,524,995	22.81%	1.30%	65.00%	5.70%
226,516,670	22.81%	1.30%	65.00%	5.70%
226,505,016	22.81%	1.30%	65.00%	5.70%
226,488,701	22.81%	1.30%	65.00%	5.70%
226,465,859	22.81%	1.30%	65.00%	5.70%
226,433,880	22.81%	1.30%	65.00%	5.70%
226,389,110	22.81%	1.30%	65.00%	5.70%
226,326,431	22.81%	1.30%	65.00%	5.70%
226,238,682	22.81%	1.30%	65.00%	5.70%
226,115,832	22.81%	1.30%	65.00%	5.70%
225,943,842	22.81%	1.30%	65.00%	5.70%
225,703,057	22.81%	1.30%	65.00%	5.70%
225,365,958	22.81%	1.30%	65.00%	5.70%
224,894,019	22.81%	1.30%	65.00%	5.70%

AIDS PROJECTIONS
Based on December
of Year Numbers
and on Present
Growth Rates and
1980 Census Data

Year - Legend		Percent Diagnosed to Not Involved This Year	Percent New Infect to Not Involved This Year	Percent Dead to Not Involved This Year	Percent Alive to Not Involved This Year
yr 1941	-------->	.00%	.00%	.00%	.00%
yr 1942	:	.00%	.00%	.00%	.00%
yr 1943	:	.00%	.00%	.00%	.00%
yr 1944	D	.00%	.00%	.00%	.00%
yr 1945	I	.00%	.00%	.00%	.00%
yr 1946	S	.00%	.00%	.00%	.00%
yr 1947	E	.00%	.00%	.00%	.00%
yr 1948	A	.00%	.00%	.00%	.00%
yr 1949	S	.00%	.00%	.00%	.00%
yr 1950	E	.00%	.00%	.00%	.00%
yr 1951	:	.00%	.00%	.00%	.00%
yr 1952	N	.00%	.00%	.00%	.00%
yr 1953	O	.00%	.00%	.00%	.00%
yr 1954	T	.00%	.00%	.00%	.00%
yr 1955	:	.00%	.00%	.00%	.00%
yr 1956	Y	.00%	.00%	.00%	.00%
yr 1957	E	.00%	.00%	.00%	.00%
yr 1958	T	.00%	.00%	.00%	.00%
yr 1959	:	.00%	.00%	.00%	.00%
yr 1960	R	.00%	.00%	.00%	.00%
yr 1961	E	.00%	.00%	.00%	.00%
yr 1962	C	.00%	.00%	.00%	.00%
yr 1963	O	.00%	.00%	.00%	.00%
yr 1964	G	.00%	.00%	.00%	.00%
yr 1965	N	.00%	.00%	.00%	.00%
yr 1966	I	.00%	.00%	.00%	.00%
yr 1967	Z	.00%	.00%	.00%	.00%
yr 1968	E	.00%	.00%	.00%	.00%
yr 1969	D	.00%	.00%	.00%	.00%
yr 1970	:	.00%	.00%	.00%	.00%
yr 1971	T	.00%	.00%	.00%	.00%
yr 1972	I	.00%	.00%	.00%	.00%
yr 1973	L	.00%	.00%	.00%	.00%
yr 1974	L	.00%	.00%	.00%	.00%
yr 1975	:	.00%	.00%	.00%	.00%
yr 1976	N	.00%	.01%	.00%	.00%
yr 1977	O	.00%	.01%	.00%	.00%
yr 1978	W	.00%	.01%	.00%	.00%
yr 1979	:	.00%	.02%	.00%	.00%
yr 1980	:	.00%	.03%	.00%	.00%
yr 1981	------->	.00%	.04%	.00%	.00%
yr 1982	Virus	.00%	.05%	.00%	.00%
yr 1983	Found	.00%	.07%	.00%	.00%
yr 1984		.00%	.10%	.00%	.01%
yr 1985		.00%	.14%	.00%	.01%
yr 1986		.00%	.19%	.00%	.01%

AIDS PROJECTIONS Based on December of Year Numbers and on Present Growth Rates and 1980 Census Data ================= Year - Legend	Percent Diagnosed to Not Involved This Year	Percent New Infect to Not Involved This Year	Percent Dead to Not Involved This Year	Percent Alive to Not Involved This Year
yr 1987	.01%	.27%	.00%	.02%
yr 1988	.01%	.38%	.00%	.02%
yr 1989	.01%	.54%	.01%	.03%
yr 1990	.02%	.76%	.01%	.04%
yr 1991	.02%	1.07%	.01%	.06%
yr 1992	.03%	1.52%	.02%	.09%
yr 1993	.04%	2.18%	.03%	.12%
yr 1994	.06%	3.16%	.04%	.18%
yr 1995	.09%	4.65%	.06%	.26%
yr 1996	.14%	7.01%	.09%	.40%
yr 1997 ------->	.22%	10.98%	.14%	.63%
yr 1998 :	.37%	18.47%	.24%	1.05%
yr 1999 :	.72%	36.01%	.47%	2.05%
yr 2000 US infect	2.24%	111.89%	1.45%	6.38%
yr 2001 :	-4.43%	-221.43%	-2.88%	-12.62%
yr 2002 :	-1.42%	-70.79%	-.92%	-4.04%
yr 2003 ------->	-.95%	-47.64%	-.62%	-2.72%
yr 2004	-.77%	-38.62%	-.50%	-2.20%
yr 2005	-.68%	-34.02%	-.44%	-1.94%
yr 2006	-.63%	-31.35%	-.41%	-1.79%
yr 2007	-.59%	-29.69%	-.39%	-1.69%
yr 2008	-.57%	-28.60%	-.37%	-1.63%
yr 2009	-.56%	-27.88%	-.36%	-1.59%
yr 2010	-.55%	-27.38%	-.36%	-1.56%
yr 2011 ------->	-.54%	-27.04%	-.35%	-1.54%
yr 2012 :	-.54%	-26.80%	-.35%	-1.53%
yr 2013 US diagno	-.53%	-26.63%	-.35%	-1.52%
yr 2014 :	-.53%	-26.51%	-.34%	-1.51%
yr 2015 ------->	-.53%	-26.42%	-.34%	-1.51%
yr 2016 :	-.53%	-26.36%	-.34%	-1.50%
yr 2017 US dead	-.53%	-26.32%	-.34%	-1.50%
yr 2018 :	-.53%	-26.29%	-.34%	-1.50%
yr 2019 ------->	-.53%	-26.27%	-.34%	-1.50%
yr 2020	-.53%	-26.25%	-.34%	-1.50%
yr 2021	-.52%	-26.24%	-.34%	-1.50%
yr 2022 ------->	-.52%	-26.23%	-.34%	-1.50%
yr 2023 :	-.52%	-26.23%	-.34%	-1.49%
yr 2024 World dia	-.52%	-26.22%	-.34%	-1.49%
yr 2025 :	-.52%	-26.22%	-.34%	-1.49%
yr 2026 ------->	-.52%	-26.22%	-.34%	-1.49%
yr 2027 :	-.52%	-26.22%	-.34%	-1.49%
yr 2028 World dea	-.52%	-26.21%	-.34%	-1.49%
yr 2029 :	-.52%	-26.21%	-.34%	-1.49%
yr 2030 ------->	-.52%	-26.21%	-.34%	-1.49%

PERCENT OF SEROPOSITIVES CONVERTING TO AIDS BY YEARS PAST INFECTION

Years Past HIV Infection	Total HTLV-III Positive Percent Becoming AIDS Diagnosed to Year	Total HTLV-III Positive Percent Remaining AIDS-Free to Year
1	5.38%	94.62%
2	10.76%	89.24%
3	16.14%	83.86%
4	21.52%	78.48%
5	26.90%	73.10%
6	32.28%	67.72%
7	37.66%	62.34%
8	43.04%	56.96%
9	48.42%	51.58%
10	53.80%	46.20%
11	59.18%	40.82%
12	64.56%	35.44%
13	69.94%	30.06%
14	75.32%	24.68%
15	80.70%	19.30%
16	86.08%	13.92%
17	91.46%	8.54%
18	96.84%	3.16%

Although not yet scientifically verified, current trend in percent of HTLV-III seropositives becoming AIDS diagnosed per year suggests the absolute lifespan of an HTLV-III seropositive individual is 21 years (+ - 1 Year) past the date of original HIV Infection.

Bibliography

"AIDS Virus: Infection Up?" *Science News* Nov. 23, 1985: 325.

Allman, W. F. "Thomas Quinn: Tracking AIDS to the Ends of the Earth." *Esquire* Dec. 1986: 211-212.

Amiel, B. "The Politics of a Killer Disease." *Maclean's* Dec. 8, 1986: 11.

Anderson, A. "Reagan Seeks Expert Advice on AIDS." *Nature* May 14, 1987: 95.

—. "Who Decides US AIDS Policy?" *Nature* May 7, 1987: 3.

Anderson, D. "AIDS: An Update on What We Know." *RN* March 1986: 50.

Barnes, D. M. "AIDS Commission bills Proliferate." *Science* 234.4793: 1136.

—. "Broad Issues Debated at AIDS Vaccine Workshop." *Science* 236.4799: 256.

—. "The Complexity of the AIDS Virus." *Science* 233.4761: 282.

—. "Keeping the AIDS Virus Out of Blood Supply." *Science* 233.4763: 515.

—. "Military Statistics on AIDS in the U.S." *Science* 233.4761: 283.

—. "Promising Results Halt Trial of Anti-AIDS Drug." *Science* 234.4772: 16.

Bazell, R. "Surviving AIDS." *The New Republic* Nov. 24, 1986: 20, 22.

Bennett, J. A. "What We Know About AIDS." *American Journal of Nursing* Sept. 1986: 1019-20.

Biner, D. "House OKs Bill Aimed at Halting AIDS Spread." *Atlanta (Georgia) Journal* Feb. 21, 1987.

Brooks, B. "Year-end Report Offers Sobering Statistics on Spread of AIDS." *Tallahassee (Florida) Democrat* Jan. 5, 1987.

Buckley, W. F. "The Buyer May Be the Smarter Person." *Moline (Illinois) Daily Dispatch* April 28, 1987: 4.

Chapman, F. S. "AIDS & Business: Problems of Costs and Compassion." *Fortune* Sept. 15, 1986: 123.

Cole, Helen M. and George D. Lundgerg, editors. "Epidemiology." *Journal of the American Medical Association* (1986): 383.

Comarow, A., et al. "The Bind That Ties All Nations." *U.S. News and World Report* Jan. 12, 1987: 64.

"Confronting AIDS: Directions for Public Health, Health Care, and Research." Washington, D.C.: National Academy Press.

Davis, L. "AIDS New Viruses to Fill in the Blanks." *Science News* 129.14: 212.

Dhundale, K. and P. M. Hubbard. "Home Care for the AIDS Patient: Safety First." *Nursing86* Sept. 1986: 34.

Dianda, M. "Grim AIDS Report." *Peninsula Times-Tribune* [Palo-Alto, California] Feb. 26, 1987.

"Doctor Wants AIDS Carriers Isolated." *Journal and Courier* Lafayette, Indiana] Jan. 1, 1987.

Encyclopedia Britannica 9: xxx.

—23: 471.

Engel, M. "Newslines From Washington." *Glamour* Jan. 1987: 110.

Gallo, R. C. "The AIDS Virus." *Scientific America* 256.1: 56.

Gunther, J. *Inside Africa.*New York: Harper and Brothers, 1955, p. 669.

Hamilton, J. O., et al. "The AIDS Epidemic and Business." *Businessweek* March 23, 1987: 123.

Hay, A. "Laboratory Safety and HIV." *The Lancet* May 9, 1987: 1094.

Houston, J. "Few Change Habits Over AIDS: Study." *Chicago (Illinois) Tribune* Feb. 19, 1987.

"Human Immunodeficiency Virus Infection in Transfusion Recipients and Their Family Members." *Morbidity and Mortality Weekly Report* 35.10: 139.

Klug, R. M. "Children With AIDS." *American Journal of Nursing* Oct. 1986: 1131.

Kuzmits, F. E. et al. "Twenty Questions About AIDS in the Workplace." *Business Horizons*, July-Aug. 1986: 37, 41.

Lacayo, R. "AIDS Goes to Court." *Time* Dec. 8, 1986: 73.

Lagone, J. "AIDS: Special Report." *Discover* 6.12: 29.

Mandel, B. *Play Safe*. Foster, California: Center for Health Information (1986): 5.

"Social Welfare Expenditures Under Public Programs." *The 1986 Information Please Almanac*(New York: Houghton Mifflin Company): 66.

Masters, W. and V. Johnson. *Human Sexuality* (Little Brown and Company) 1985.

May, R. M., et al. "Transmission Dynamics of HIV Infection." *Nature* March 12, 1987: 137.

Mecklin, J. "Houston Biologist Investigated Over AIDS Vaccine." *Houston (Texas) Post* March 6, 1987.

Norman, C. "Sex and Needles, Not Insects and Pigs, Spread AIDS in Florida Town." *Science* 234.4775: 416.

"The Panic Spreads." *The Economist* Nov. 15, 1986: 70.

Parkins, A. "Insurers Want AIDS Treated Equally." *Capital Times*[Madison, Wisconsin] Jan. 8, 1987.

Petit, C. "California to Vote on AIDS Proposition." *Science* 234.4774: 277.

Price, J. "Leading AIDS Scientist Sees No Cure in 'Anyone's Lifetime.'" *Washington (D.C.) Times* March 26, 1987.

—. "Public Besieged by 'Drugs' That Don't Work." *Washington (D.C.) Times* Feb. 24, 1987.

"Science and the Citizen." *Scientific American* Jan. 1987: 58-59.

Scitovsky, A. A., et al. "Estimates of the Direct and Indirect Costs of Acquired Immunodeficiency Syndrome in the United States, 1985, 1986, and 1991." *Public Health Reports* 102.1: 8.

Seabrook, C. "Reagan OKs AIDS Education Plan." *Journal* [Atlanta, Georgia], Feb. 26, 1987.

Serrill, Michael S. "In the Grip Of the Scourge." *Time* Feb. 16, 1987: 58.

Shuit, D. "Fourfold Increase in AIDS Medical Costs is Expected by 1991." *Los Angeles (California) Times* Feb. 26, 1987.

Siwolop, S., et al. "AIDS Research: Where the Battle Stands." *Businessweek* March 23, 1987: 130.

Smilgis, M. "The Big Chill: Fear of AIDS." *Time* Feb. 16, 1987: 56.

Smith, R. "AIDS Policy Called Too Little, Too Late." *Akron (Ohio) Beacon Journal*, Jan. 31, 1987.

"Social Welfare Expenditures Under Public Programs." *The 1986 Information Please Almanac* (New York: Houghton Mifflin Company), p. 66.

Stoller, B. "AIDS." *The Journal of Practical Nursing* Dec. 1985: 26-30.

"Volunteers, Home Care, and Money: How San Francisco Has Mobilized." *Business Week* March 23, 1987: 125.

Wallis, C. "You Haven't Heard Anything Yet." *Time* Feb. 16, 1987: 54, 56.

Whelan, E. M. "Wishful Thinking About an Epidemic." *Across the Board* Oct. 1986: 34.

Subject Index

Name Index